MW00620114

Design and cover art by Armen Khudgaryan.

Disclaimer:

End Insomnia LLC is not a healthcare entity and does not practice medicine or offer mental health services. Its programs, suggestions, and other offerings are informational and educational in nature and do not diagnose, treat, prevent, or cure any medical condition or replace competent licensed medical advice. All references to assisting in the alleviation of insomnia or its symptoms hold common English-language meanings, such as "restore," "resolve," "heal," "alleviate," "help," "assist," "end," etc. None of these terms are used or may be interpreted to signify any medical or mental health activity for which a license is required.

End Insomnia LLC does not guarantee that its approaches or programs solve 100% of every person's insomnia. Some insomnia is caused by factors such as: hormone imbalance, severe emotional trauma, physical pain, and medications that can only be resolved through medical or other treatment. And while the program offered by End Insomnia has helped many people return to normal and healthy sleep patterns, it does not guarantee particular results. However, your success will be greatly determined by your diligence and compliance with the program.

"

"Out of suffering have emerged the strongest souls; the most massive characters are seared with scars."

— KHALIL GIBRAN

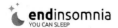

Contents

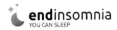

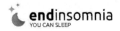

A NOTE FOR SHIFT WORKERS AND OTHERS WITH ATYPICAL SCHEDULES

To keep things simple for the greatest number of people, I wrote this book assuming "typical" sleep/awake schedules—therefore, terms such as "night" and "day" are used accordingly.

If you are a shift worker—or your schedule otherwise fluctuates—you may not be able to apply these guidelines exactly as directed. Do your best with the schedule constraints you have.

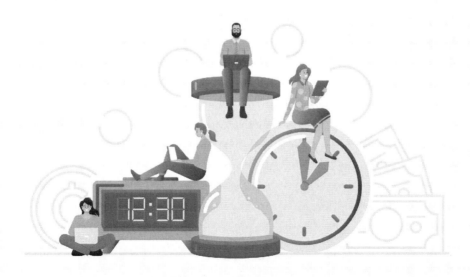

Introduction

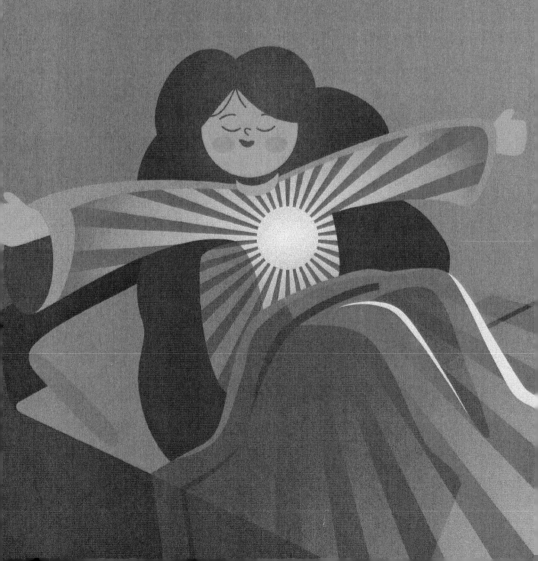

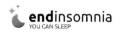

You have insomnia—persistent difficulty falling asleep or staying a sleep through the night. Insomnia often results in significant distress during the day and night and makes it hard to function or feel like yourself. While many people experience short-term insomnia, for some, it sticks around and can come to dominate their lives. Insomnia is often considered a long-term issue if it lasts longer than three months.

Insomnia is an awful experience that can come to dominate your life. Many struggling with sleep try everything to fix it and remain stuck. The lack of sustainable solutions to permanently overcome insomnia can leave those suffering from it exhausted, confused, and enormously frustrated.

This book will offer you a new solution, the **End Insomnia System**. This system offers a permanent path out of insomnia.

Derived from extensive research and experimentation, the End Insomnia System pulls together the best tools and resources from multiple evidence-based approaches to insomnia and psychological change in general (most notably Acceptance and Commitment Therapy).

This new system is designed to *target and overcome the root cause of insomnia.* It aims to equip you with the knowledge and tools to take back your sleep and maintain better sleep for life.

If your experience of insomnia is anything like that of people who have benefitted from this approach, you might relate to the following:

+ Your nights are filled with desperate, futile attempts to make yourself sleep.

+ The consequences of awful sleep plague your days: exhaustion, brain fog, and anxiety about the night to come.

+ You stress over how you can possibly have a good life in the future when you are consistently sleeping poorly.

+ Sleep and insomnia weigh heavily on your mind, and you worry about the long-term health effects of living like this

+ Your sleep problems leave you feeling enormously frustrated, alone, and overwhelmed, and you feel like you're "never going to sleep again".

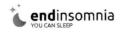

+ You keep trying to force sleep to happen which puts an incredible amount of pressure and makes the situation even worse.

+ You think your insomnia is "unique" and something "must be wrong" with you

+ Insomnia has made it hard to be the person you want to be.

+ You obsessively google for 'the solution' only to find unhelpful articles and feel like a "failure."

+ You feel trapped in insomnia and are unsure if there is hope for you to ever move past it because EVERYTHING you've tried has failed.

That sense of "I've tried everything, but nothing works" is very common. Many people have found that the mainstream approaches to insomnia do not work for them.

These protocols are often based on faulty assumptions about the problem, so their advice on how to fix it can be ineffective.

If you've felt like you've tried everything under the sun to fix your insomnia and nothing has worked, this book will explain why—and teach you what to do instead.

Once you have a new understanding of *why* you can't sleep, this book will present a comprehensive system to help you **permanently end your insomnia.** This solution is radically different from everything you may have tried before, including:

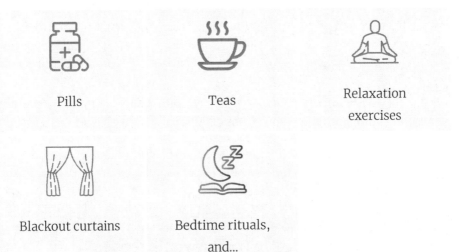

Pills

Teas

Relaxation exercises

Blackout curtains

Bedtime rituals, and...

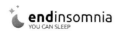

...well, countless other quick fixes—and even the supposed "gold standard" of insomnia treatment, Cognitive Behavioral Therapy for insomnia (CBT-i).

These approaches often focus on doing things to try to make sleep happen. I'll show you why that doesn't work long term.

Rather than trying to *make* sleep happen, the End Insomnia System is a long-term approach that focuses on *resolving the factors that **stop** you from sleeping.*

So, even if you believe you've exhausted all your options, there is hope. By the end of this book, my goal is for you to be far along on your journey to great sleep.

In Part 1 of this book, I'll share the story of how and why I created the End Insomnia System. You will also take several self-assessments to examine the current state of your insomnia and get a sense of the changes you will likely experience if you apply the knowledge and skills in this book. I will address common doubts and objections that you might have.

I will ensure you have accurate information about what's really going on with your sleep—and with your insomnia.

We'll do a deep dive into why nothing you've tried to fix your insomnia has worked—and I'll give you evidence to support the central point of this book:

> To overcome insomnia, you need to calm the sleep-related anxiety and associated nervous system hyperarousal that fuels your sleep issues.

A variety of causes can bring on insomnia, but long-term insomnia is generally maintained by sleep anxiety and chronic nervous system activation at night.

While overcoming these factors might seem like a near-insurmountable task, Part 2 of this book will show you exactly how to achieve that.

I'll let you in on a little secret: *There are only two forces that control sleep.* You'll find out what they are in Chapter 4—and throughout Part 2, you'll learn how to get them to work for you so you can move toward better sleep.

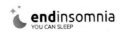

In **Part 2** of the book, you'll learn the entire framework that I call the **End Insomnia System**.

The End Insomnia System combines:

+ An eye-opening set of knowledge to bring relief, understanding, and hope to your situation.

+ Gentle and sustainable guidelines for increasing your body's natural tendency to fall and stay asleep.

+ A complete set of psychological tools for managing your distress and lowering your anxiety over time, including mindfulness, acceptance, self-compassion, and powerful ways to work with distressing thoughts.

+ Specific guidance for what to do at night when you can't sleep in order to move toward a long-term insomnia solution.

+ A framework for approaching days when you feel fatigued so that you suffer less, live more fully and lower your "performance anxiety" around sleep.

+ Ways to be kinder to yourself—especially as you work through overcoming your insomnia. Insomnia is hard!

+ A daily practice to recondition your mind and nervous system to be calmer in situations that have typically sparked anxiety.

+ A set of empowering mindsets and attitudes that you can lean on when you are suffering that will propel you forward toward good sleep.

+ Guidance on how to find a support system that will genuinely help you (and won't inadvertently undermine your hard work).

In **Part 3,** we'll make sure you are clear on how to navigate the journey to better sleep—and what to expect along the way.

By the end of this book, you'll see how all of these pieces fit together to empower you to overcome your ingrained sleep anxiety and permanently end your insomnia.

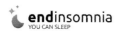
Just remember: It's not enough to simply have an intellectual understanding of this system. You must apply the exercises and guidelines in this book to experience real change.

Many have turned their sleep around with this system. I believe you can, too.

THE CENTRAL IDEA
OF THIS BOOK:

As long as you have entrenched *anxiety about insomnia*, you will struggle to improve your sleep in a lasting way. To end insomnia, you need to calm the anxiety that drives it.

Rather than trying to make sleep happen, your focus must be on reducing your anxiety about insomnia and its consequences. As we'll explore in this book, when you're stuck in a loop of anxiety about your sleep, your nervous system makes it very hard for you to sleep.

As you lessen your anxiety over time, your nervous system will settle down, and sleep will begin to happen for you without effort.

Although there are many ups and downs in the journey of overcoming insomnia, as you reduce your anxiety layer by layer, you will transform your mind and attain great sleep for life.

The **End Insomnia System** will show you how.

Before we jump in, let's cover a few scenarios where this system may not be the right fit for you.

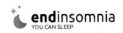

This Book *May Not* Be for You If:

Your sleep issues are *primarily* driven by a current stressor unrelated to sleep.

If you are under chronic stress about something—such as work, family, relationships, or past trauma—and you're aware that your stress about that issue is specifically the thing that keeps you awake at night, then it may be more effective for you to focus on addressing the current problem. Working with a therapist can be a great option to help with that.

Alternatively, if your sleep issues are caused directly by pain or other symptoms of illness (such as cancer) or hormonal changes (as with menopause), then the best course of action is to work to address or alleviate the underlying issue, if possible. Insomnia can also sometimes be a side effect of certain medications, which this system is not designed to address directly.

In all of these instances, the End Insomnia System may still be helpful for three reasons:

First, even if a life situation may have triggered the sleep issues when poor sleep drags on for a while, it's easy to start developing some anxiety about sleep that reinforces your insomnia. This book can help you better manage and overcome the extra sleep anxiety that may be compounding the issues you are facing and making it harder to sleep.

Second, this book will give you strategies to increase your chances of getting better sleep, even if you're dealing with other stressors that make it harder to sleep.

Third, the strategies in this book for managing difficult thoughts and feelings and for finding more peace in situations that you don't have full control over can be generalized to anything. These strategies can help you find more calm and deal more effectively with whatever stressor you may be facing.

Also, if you find your sleep troubles continue after the original issue that brought them on is resolved—or if you start to find your anxieties more centered on sleep itself—then the knowledge and tools in this book will help.

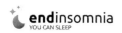
This Book Is *Not* for You If:

1. **YOU NEED SLEEP APNEA TREATMENT.**

    Sleep apnea is a physiological condition in which a person's breathing repeatedly stops and starts during the night. If you have sleep apnea, you may wake up gasping for air during the night. Loud snoring is another common symptom.

    People with sleep apnea often report that they don't have trouble sleeping, but they feel fatigued and unrefreshed during the day, even when they think they've slept a normal amount. **Sleep apnea is a condition that should be treated by a medical professional.** A physician can order a sleep study if you suspect you might have sleep apnea.

    HOWEVER: If you are getting treatment for sleep apnea but also have insomnia, then it's likely this book will help.

2. **YOU ARE LOOKING FOR A QUICK FIX—AND EXPECT AN INSTANT, MAGICAL SOLUTION FOR YOUR INSOMNIA.**

    Alas: Overcoming insomnia takes work—and time. I'd offer you a quick fix if I could, but there are no quick fixes for insomnia that actually work. You'll learn more about this in the chapters to come.

    The End Insomnia System takes time to learn and requires perseverance. You need to apply the system to get results. And you need to understand that ups and downs are an inevitable part of the process.

    If you can take a long-term view and remain committed to the practices and perspectives offered by this system, then this system IS for you—and you CAN leave your insomnia behind.

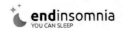

Moving Forward To A Life of Better Sleep

The system you learn here—the End Insomnia System—will not just give you a way to resolve your insomnia and enjoy great sleep.

It will radically change your relationship with your thoughts and emotions, and it will teach you empowering ways to find greater ease and resilience in all areas of your life.

I wrote this book to show you how you can resolve your insomnia **on your own**—but you don't have to.

If you read this book and decide you'd like help reversing insomnia **as fast and easily as possible,** we have designed the End Insomnia Program to give you guidance and support through implementing everything you're about to learn.

The End Insomnia Program offers:

✦ Over 6 hours of premium video footage with detailed presentations.

✦ Accountability and expert guidance by trained sleep coaches.

✦ A supportive community for fresh insights and inspiration.

✦ Additional tools, workbooks, and resources to take your learning deeper.

VISIT THE LINK BELOW TO LEARN MORE:

https://endinsomnia.com/program

To better sleep and a well-rested life,

Ivo

Part 1

Targeting the Root Cause of Insomnia: Why What You've Tried Doesn't Work —And What *DOES*

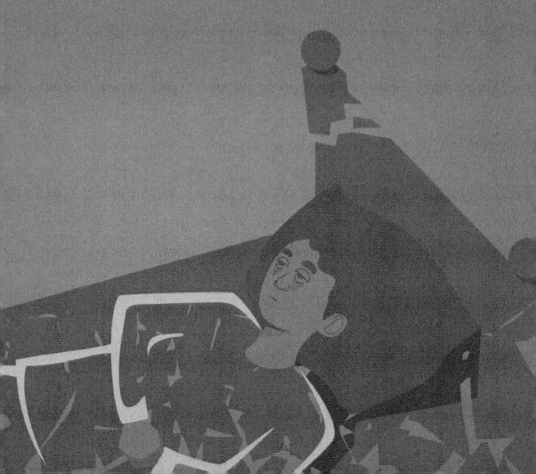

CHAPTER 1

Why I Believe This System Can Help You— When Nothing You've Tried Has Worked

Whether you've turned to doctors, therapists, or internet sources to get help with your sleep, it's common to be left feeling like the people you're turning to for help don't truly get what you're going through.

I'm not one of those people.

The approach you'll learn about in this book emerged directly from my own multi-year struggle with insomnia. While the system was refined through helping others overcome insomnia, I created it because I desperately needed to do something to help myself after I had exhausted all other options.

I now want to share the story of my descent into insomnia—and how I resolved it. My intention in sharing this is to help you believe that I

1. Know what the experience of insomnia is truly like, and

2. Know how to truly resolve this.

My insomnia started after a particularly stressful period in my life. The stress came and went... but my sleepless nights stayed.

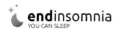

So I slogged through days feeling tense and dog-tired all the time like my body was made of cement. My mind was dominated by brain fog, stress, and worry that this would go on forever.

There was no escape from feeling anxious about what my sleep would be like the next night... and how it would make me feel the next day.

At first, I desperately hoped my insomnia would work itself out, but...

As the months went on, my insomnia only got *worse*.

I'd lay awake for hours. Just as I'd fall asleep, my brain would jerk awake in the middle of the night. I would constantly toss and turn in bed... and it seemed impossible to relax my body and mind.

Sometimes my heart would pound as I climbed into bed, getting worse as the minutes passed.

I felt like my body had betrayed me. Like there was something wrong with me... and my ability to sleep was broken. Soon, I started doubting that I could consistently get a good night's rest ever again.

Insomnia was ruining every part of my life.

Even the things that used to bring me joy felt empty. I started avoiding my friends, social gatherings and even talking to people altogether. I didn't have the energy or mood for any of it, and it seemed like no one could understand what I was going through.

I felt like I was failing in life and that I just couldn't be the person I wanted to be. It seemed impossible to live well.

So I tried virtually everything to ease my insomnia.

I spent a huge amount of time Googling for the solution. And convincing myself the latest 'shiny object' would *have to be it*.

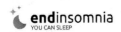

And I spent a small fortune on so-called "solutions." To name a few, I tried...

+ Sleeping pills

+ Sleep hygiene

+ Herbal teas

+ Bedtime rituals

+ Blackout curtains

+ A weighted blanket

+ Pre-bedtime exercise and relaxation routines

+ Carefully timed hot showers

+ Quitting caffeine and alcohol

+ All kinds of so-called "sleep hacks"

+ Cutting out water and liquids four hours before bed

+ Staying away from screens and blue light before bed

+ Getting a lot of sun in the morning (I thought, *"the problem must be low Vitamin D levels!"*)

+ B12 supplements and shots (*"No, wait... the real problem is B12 deficiency!"*)

+ And much more

These solutions either didn't work at all—or they failed to provide lasting relief.

I even saw a specialist in Cognitive Behavioral Therapy for insomnia (CBT-i)— the so-called "gold standard" for insomnia treatment.

I pinned all my hopes on it working, and while it helped me get rest for a few weeks, my dreadful sleep and anxiety came back after I stopped seeing the therapist.

I was back at square one... and couldn't go on like this.

So I dedicated myself to finding a permanent solution for insomnia that actually works.

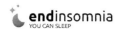

I obsessively poured through all the latest studies on sleep and insomnia.

Eventually, I stumbled on research that revealed while insomnia is often triggered by stress, it's *maintained* by sleep anxiety.

And the more we approach nighttime worried about sleeplessness and its daytime consequences, the more **the nervous system becomes conditioned to automatically enter a hyperaroused, "fight or flight" mode.** These findings were recently confirmed by Stanford University researchers.

Suddenly it made sense why all the conventional solutions for insomnia failed to provide permanent relief for myself and so many people.

Little to none of the existing treatments work to directly end sleep anxiety, calm the nervous system, or undo the conditioned hyperarousal at the root of insomnia.

Instead, they work more like temporary "BandAid" solutions.

So I took this information and set out to create a new method. One that actually resolves the root cause of stress-triggered insomnia.

First, I teamed up with a therapist who specializes in insomnia. He wanted a more effective and lasting way to help his clients escape sleeplessness, and I just wanted to sleep normally and enjoy life again.

Together, we dug through the latest research on anxiety, hyperarousal, and psychological change.

We knew we were onto something when we looked into a relatively new, clinically-proven therapy. A treatment that's been shown to reduce the symptoms of anxiety and hyperarousal in human clinical trials. Yet strangely, this approach had hardly been used on insomnia.

It's called **Acceptance and Commitment Therapy (ACT)**, and only recently has it started to get the attention it deserves:

Psychology Today reported that "ACT is rapidly growing in influence and popularity and meta-studies have found that it is as least as effective as Cognitive-Behavioral Therapy."

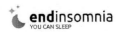

And Baylor College of Medicine, one of the top-ranked medical institutions in the United States, only further confirmed our suspicions that ACT could be a breakthrough in insomnia treatment.

They reported:

"Changing one's relationship to anxiety, from struggle to acceptance, has the paradoxical effect of reducing anxiety symptoms, to the same extent or more than traditional, cognitive behavioral approaches, as suggested by large randomized clinical trials of ACT."

Yet as we discovered an ever-growing body of research that suggests ACT could be effective at treating insomnia, I wondered, **"How does struggling against this dreadful experience—and trying to control the parts of it that I can't control—lead to ongoing insomnia?"**

What we found was that distressing thoughts, and especially how we react to such thoughts, can trigger the same survival response in the brain and body that occurs if we are in physical danger. Simply by thinking something like "What if I get terrible sleep again tonight? I can't stand another day of this!" and then beginning to fixate on and obsess about that thought, your body floods with stress hormones and anxiety.

That's why ACT can calm sleep anxiety and reverse conditioned hyperarousal. It helps you change the way you respond to the dreadful thoughts, feelings, and physical sensations you get from not sleeping. When you respond with less struggle, more acceptance, and adopt new, empowering perspectives, your nervous system can begin to calm down.

However, I remained stuck when we tried to put the existing ACT treatment guidelines into practice. We found the existing treatment guidelines unclear, confusing, and very hard to follow.

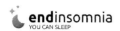

Fortunately, we had the expertise in mental health to clarify and expand on existing ACT techniques. We then added additional tools and perspectives from other schools of psychology to address the other factors contributing to sleep anxiety.

I tested our findings on myself to see what actually helped. And after months of experimentation, research and analysis, we completed the first version of the End Insomnia System... and what happened next felt like a miracle.

When I applied these new methods, my sleep anxiety started getting weaker. Within a few weeks, I felt calmer during the day. I was at ease at night—even if I didn't sleep. Within the first three months, I felt a dramatic difference. And a few months after that, I was sleeping well consistently!

Next, we tested the approach with a diverse range of clients and refined it.

When we saw how well it worked for other insomniacs—many who had been struggling for years, or even decades—I knew we had to share this approach with others who shared the same pain as I did.

The rest of this book is dedicated to showing you the exact method that has now helped hundreds of people end insomnia for good.

This journey started because I needed a solution so badly myself.

I'm happy to report that today, I'm totally free from the shackles of insomnia. I never worry about sleep—it just happens effortlessly. I wake up rested, refreshed, and energetic.

And on the (very rare) nights I don't sleep as well, I feel calm and accepting. My work productivity is through the roof, and I finally have the energy to be present with my friends and family. I'm truly back to living a full life.

I am free, and hundreds of others have used these principles to achieve similar results. And now you can, too.

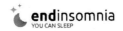

Self-Assessment:
The Current State of Your Insomnia

There are a lot of ways insomnia can manifest, so let's check in with YOUR experience. Here's a brief self-assessment to evaluate the current state of your insomnia.

Below, rate yourself on a scale from 0–4 on how accurate the statements are, 0 means "not true for me at all," and 4 means "very true for me."

Once you've filled in a rating for each statement, total up your numbers and use the scoring key below the self-assessment to get more insight into your specific situation.

INSOMNIA CHECK-IN STATEMENT	SELF EATING
1. I have trouble getting to sleep or staying asleep, despite doing everything I can to try to help myself sleep better.	
2. I feel deeply frustrated when, once again, I find myself unable to sleep—when sleep is what I want more than anything.	
3. My body seems to betray me at night. I experience things like an increased heart rate, sudden "jerks" just as I'm falling asleep, racing thoughts, or a sense of panic. I generally feel like my ability to fall asleep or stay asleep is broken.	
4. I often get up in the morning feeling totally depleted and dreading the day to come.	

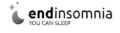

5. My worries about sleep often weigh on my mind during the day.

6. I feel fatigue and physical discomfort during the day that is hard to bear.

7. As night approaches, I feel on edge, knowing I may be in for yet another hard night.

8. I feel powerless over my insomnia and trapped in a cycle of misery that doesn't seem to have an end.

9. I have tried all kinds of things (pills, relaxation techniques, distraction, CBT-i, bedtime rituals, sleep hygiene, etc.) to try to improve my sleep, but nothing works long term.

10. At times, my anxious thoughts feel like my worst enemy.

11. I am afraid that I will have insomnia for the rest of my life and that it will significantly affect my health.

12. Insomnia holds me back from being the person I want to be.

13. I fear that my sleep issues may cause me to fail or be inadequate in my responsibilities (for example, as a parent, spouse, professional, student, or friend).

14. I feel alone in my experience of insomnia and misunderstood by others who don't struggle with sleep.

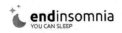

INSOMNIA CHECK-IN STATEMENT	SELF EATING

15. I feel grief about the presence of insomnia in my life and all that it has taken from me.

16. I have withdrawn from activities or hold myself back from my aspirations because I don't feel in a state to live the life I want to live.

17. My insomnia makes it hard to travel, sleep away from home, or commit to plans or exciting opportunities.

18. I am trapped in a situation that often feels traumatic, and I am desperate for a way out.

19. Insomnia is one of the worst things—maybe the worst thing—that has ever happened to me.

20. I am reluctant to get my hopes up about a new approach to overcoming insomnia because I've been let down so many times.

TOTAL UP YOUR SCORE:

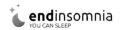
■ What Your Score Means

Score: 55–80

Lost in Insomnia

You are experiencing a great deal of suffering from insomnia. Your attempts to help yourself have left you disappointed, and you likely feel trapped and overwhelmed by insomnia. Your nights are often miserable, and your days are hard to get through. Insomnia is a restricting and limiting force in your life. It may seem there is no end in sight, even though you are longing for change.

The good news is that all of these experiences can be reversed. Additionally, because you are in such great pain, it means you likely have a lot of incentive to learn a new approach to insomnia and apply it long term.

The knowledge and practices within the End Insomnia System can make a world of difference for you if you apply them in a patient and persistent way. You will also likely get a good dose of initial relief from simply learning what this book teaches you about what is going on with your sleep, why your efforts to help yourself have failed, and why you feel so trapped.

While it may be hard to imagine how you'll get from your current state to consistent great sleep, if you approach the information in this book with an open mind and a willingness to make big changes, you can sleep well again.

Score: 30–54

Managing but Suffering

If your score is in this range, it means you've found ways to tolerate some of the difficulties that come with insomnia. Perhaps you've been able to still live your life and get by, but the burden of insomnia is still great.

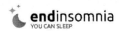

You likely feel held back from being the person you want to be, and insomnia is never far from your mind. You still experience the pervasive distress of insomnia, day and night.

Using the End Insomnia System as a framework to understand and address your insomnia in a new way will be a relief for you. As you apply this system, you'll become even more resilient to the experience of insomnia and learn a whole set of new knowledge and skills to lay the groundwork for a return to great sleep.

With consistent practice, you can remove the anxiety that fuels insomnia layer by layer and begin to regain trust in your natural ability to sleep. Full reversal of insomnia awaits if you apply this system.

Score: 0–29
Finding Resilience and Ready to Take Your Sleep to the Next Level

You've found ways to be resilient in the face of poor sleep, and your life is not dominated by insomnia.

This is excellent. You may have found other tools to work through your sleep-related anxiety or naturally feel confident in your ability to function on however much sleep you get.

However, you may feel you have plateaued in your journey out of insomnia and are not yet where you'd like to be with your sleep. You may have specific sticking points related to insomnia that you find persistent and hard to overcome.

The End Insomnia System will fill in gaps in your understanding and equip you with specific practices and mindsets to apply to the areas where you are stuck.

With a little help, you are not far away from addressing the root of your insomnia so that you can enjoy great sleep for the rest of your days.

KEY CHAPTER TAKEAWAYS

☑ If you struggle with sleep—are frustrated by being unable to sleep at night and plagued by sleep anxiety during the day—you are not alone.

☑ While insomnia is difficult to bear, equipped with a proper understanding, appropriate skills, and a commitment to the long-term journey of overcoming insomnia, you *can* sleep well again.

CHAPTER 2

Addressing Common Doubts and Objections

In the introduction, we talked about some of the reasons the system might not be for you—for example, having sleep apnea or wanting a magical quick fix. Now let's talk about some reasons you might think the system is not for you—when in fact, it really might be.

OBJECTION 1

You're saying anxiety is the cause of insomnia. But I have insomnia, and I'm not anxious.

Maybe the term "anxiety" is getting in the way. Instead, think of your *physical sensations.*

What's going on in your body at night when you can't sleep? Or when you wake in the middle of the night? Do you feel wired, agitated, or frustrated? Is your heart pounding? Are your muscles tense, ready to spring into action? Are your thoughts racing?

This is a textbook description of a fight-or-flight survival response. This physiological response follows directly from perceiving a possible threat to your physical or mental well-being. Anxiety is another word for this experience.

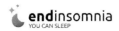

Anxiety is a term that most people with insomnia identify with. Anxiety (and the physiological response that comes with it) arises when something we encounter evokes fear and uncertainty. Having persistent sleep issues, and having to deal with the consequences, typically involves both fear and uncertainty.

(If you don't relate to the term "anxiety," that's okay: I'm really talking about the physiological experience that makes it hard to sleep.)

Ask yourself: How different would insomnia be if you were truly unafraid of the consequences of not sleeping? If you had no concerns about sleep—or the lack of it—during the day or night?

If you weren't anxious about having insomnia, would insomnia really be an issue?

OBJECTION 2

I've been disappointed so many times. Why should I believe in this?

Many people with insomnia have tried so many things to help themselves and have been disappointed again and again—so they are often slow to put their hope in anything new. If that's you, I get it. You can only be disappointed so many times before you begin to carry skepticism toward anyone who says they have the solution.

However, the End Insomnia System differs from mainstream approaches in that it identifies and targets the anxiety underlying insomnia, rather than targeting sleep itself. It offers a comprehensive set of tools and information that work together to "unlearn" your sleep anxiety—which can be done if approached with a willingness to stay the course for the long term.

Insomnia is painful and uncomfortable as it is, and you have little to lose by committing yourself to the system described in this book, even if it takes time to deliver results. (We'll get into the specific phases of the journey out of insomnia and discuss the timeline for this process later in the book.)

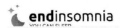

OBJECTION 3:

I think my brain or body is broken and won't let me
sleep, so I don't know if this can help me.

You might believe this system won't work for you because something is "broken"
inside of you that prevents you from sleeping. It's easy to feel broken as you lie
wide awake for hours and hours in a state of agitation—and it seems everyone
you know is enjoying great sleep. These sorts of beliefs can take a deeper hold
when you are exposed to inaccurate information, such as reading random online
forums or self-help articles written by people who don't know what they are
talking about.

You might also think there is something physically wrong with you that
triggers any strange physical symptoms you experience at night, like suddenly
"jerking" awake just as you're falling asleep.

You are not broken. As you'll learn in Chapter 4, you cannot lose the ability to sleep.

It is possible, however, for sleep-related anxiety and nervous system arousal
to get in the way of sleep happening. The strange physical symptoms you
experience at night, which might leave you feeling like your body is betraying
you, are just signs of your nervous system going into fight-or-flight mode.

This can all be unlearned. When you address the anxiety and nervous system
arousal, things will change for you.

OBJECTION 4:

I worry my insomnia is too unique for this to help me.

You might believe that this system can work for some people... but not for you,
because you have a unique experience of insomnia. While insomnia can show

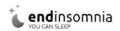

up in different ways, and even though the exact sleep struggles may vary from person to person, the core issues and the solutions are almost always the same.

It can be a relief to realize that the experience of insomnia that has caused you so much distress and left you feeling so alone is an experience shared by millions of people worldwide.

You are not alone. And you are not stuck with insomnia forever.

 ## OBJECTION 5:

I worry my psychology is too unique for this to help me.

I also sometimes hear people express the concern that, even if their insomnia is not unique, perhaps their psychological makeup is—and therefore, this system can't work for them.

It's true that you are unique. That doesn't mean this system cannot help you.

The knowledge and ACT-based tools in this system can help improve the sleep of people who may also have various forms of OCD, ADHD, a history of trauma, pre-existing anxiety or depression... and all sorts of other unique life histories.

(However, it's important to note that the system in this book is *specifically aimed at reversing insomnia*, not addressing these other conditions.)

■ Ready to Try Something New?

As you progress through this book, bring an open mind and a willingness to try new things. Even if, up to this point, you've believed you are broken or beyond help, if you apply yourself to the practices and knowledge contained in these pages and are patient and committed through the long-term process, you can end your insomnia.

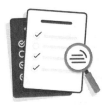

KEY CHAPTER TAKEAWAYS

☑ If you feel beyond help, I urge you to give this system a chance. It is a long-term approach and is likely different from anything you've tried before.

☑ Your body and brain are not broken, and your insomnia is not uniquely unsolvable. If you address the anxiety and other factors that keep your insomnia going, you will sleep. Even if you deal with other factors that make it harder to sleep, reducing your sleep anxiety will help to improve your situation.

CHAPTER 3

What's Really Going On With Your Sleep

People with insomnia work very hard to not be people with insomnia. By the time someone comes to this system, they generally feel they have tried everything.

People with insomnia are exhausted—but they certainly aren't lazy. The amount of time, effort, and money they have spent is often astonishing.

I want to show you why the things you've tried to fix your insomnia haven't worked—and give you a new path to end your insomnia for good.

First, we need to give you some foundational, accurate information about sleep—and about insomnia. There is an enormous amount of misinformation out there. Without the right understanding of what's happening to you, you can't address the core problem.

This chapter will explore what's really going on.

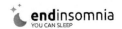

The Science of Sleep

There is a tremendous amount of sleep research—but only a few key things you need to know. Here are the basics about sleep stages and sleep cycles:

■ Sleep Stages

Each night, a person repeatedly cycles through various stages of sleep. These are:

+ Awake
+ Very light sleep
+ Light sleep
+ Deep sleep
+ REM sleep

A hypnogram is a graph made by monitoring a person's sleep over the course of a night. It shows the sleep stages the sleeper passes through.

Here's a hypnogram that shows a night of a typical adult sleeper:

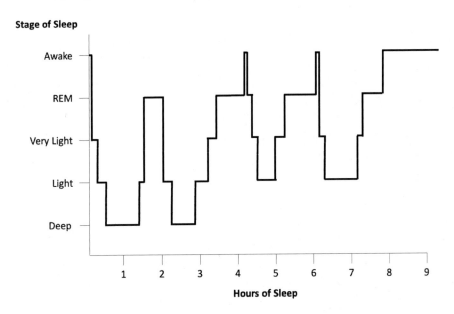

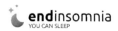

Very Light Sleep:

From being awake, you first enter into very light sleep. This occurs as you lie down at night, even though you may still feel awake. The body begins to relax, and the brain begins to slow down. This is the stage where some people experience "hypnic jerks" (those twitches that wake you just as you're falling asleep).

Light Sleep:

Falling deeper into sleep, you enter into light sleep. In light sleep, your brain and body continue to slow down and are in a more restful state.

As much as 50–60% of the night is spent in very light or light sleep.

Deep Sleep:

Deep sleep is the most restorative phase: Your brain activity is at its lowest, and your body completes various repairs on itself.

Only about 15–20% of the night is spent in deep sleep. As we get older, we tend to sleep more lightly and spend less time in deep sleep. You are less likely to be woken up in deep sleep, but you may feel dazed for a few minutes if you are.

 IMPORTANT:

As you can see from the hypnogram above, *you get your deepest—and most restorative—sleep during the first part of your time asleep.*

REM Sleep:

Rapid eye movement (REM) sleep occurs primarily in the second half of your night. Your brain is more active in REM sleep, and your heart rate and breathing rate are higher. Most dreaming also occurs in this sleep stage. It's easier to be woken up in this stage because your body is closer to wakefulness. You will often feel groggy when woken from REM sleep.

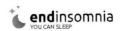

Sleep Cycles

Each night, your body goes through multiple **sleep cycles** in which you pass through the various sleep stages. People typically pass through *four to five sleep cycles per night*, each lasting for about 90 to 120 minutes.

At the end of each sleep cycle, there is a **brief awakening.** Most people don't remember these awakenings the following day, but they are a normal part of sleeping. They give you a chance to use the toilet or shift position for comfort. (These awakenings may be an evolutionary legacy, as they provide an opportunity to check for danger during the night.)

■ What to Remember About Sleep Stages

When you have insomnia, there are two key things to remember about sleep stages. First, it's normal to wake up multiple times, and these awakenings happen more often in the latter part of the night—when sleep is lighter. When you have insomnia and experience these normal awakenings, rather than quickly re-entering sleep, you might realize that you're awake and begin to consciously or unconsciously feel alarmed about being awake, wondering whether or not you will fall back to sleep.

The way to deal with nighttime awakenings is to normalize them: Remind yourself it's okay and natural to wake up at night. Nothing is wrong with you if you experience this, and it doesn't need to cause panic. With time, as you become more accepting of when you are awake and less alarmed by insomnia, you will come to experience these awakenings without a strong reaction and will be able to re-enter into sleep like a normal sleeper.

Second, if you get at least some sleep, you're likely getting most of the deepest and most restorative stage of sleep, which happens during the first part of your time asleep and is enough to get by on.

Sleep researchers sometimes refer to the minimum amount of sleep your body needs to function in the day as "core sleep." How much core sleep a person needs to function varies from about 3−5 hours.

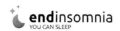

When you get your core sleep, you are getting almost all of your deep sleep, and usually a good portion of other sleep stages as well. This is enough to function during the day, even if you don't feel good and would prefer to get more sleep. If it seems as though you're barely sleeping at all, but you are still able to stay awake through the day, it's likely you're actually getting the core sleep your body needs to get by.

Although running on only core sleep isn't fun, it's a part of life sometimes and doesn't have dire consequences. Examples of people who often just get core sleep for extended periods of time include many doctors and medical residents, certain military personnel, parents who are often up with a new baby, and long-distance boat racers.

On the topic of getting your core sleep, it's also worth knowing that a substantial body of research shows that people with insomnia often misperceive and underestimate the amount of sleep they actually get. [,,]

In part, this is because people with insomnia are often influenced by negative beliefs and expectations, which then affect their perceptions regarding their sleep.

Additionally, research has shown that when people with insomnia are woken from light or REM stages of sleep, they often report that they had not been asleep at all—even though the laboratory equipment measuring their sleep proved this was not the case. [,]

When you're tired, groggy, and have an aroused nervous system in the middle of the night, it can be hard to accurately perceive how long you've been awake or whether or not you have slept.

So, there is good reason to think that your sleep may not be as bad as you perceive it to be, which can be a relief.

Knowing this can help you feel less alarmed and threatened if you don't get much sleep. The story you tell yourself about how bad your situation is matters, and these facts about sleep stages can help you tell yourself a less scary story.

That's sleep. What about insomnia? How—and why—does it develop?

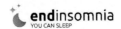

The Science of Insomnia

Insomnia develops in a predictable way for almost everyone, due to combined:

+ Risk factors
+ Triggering event
+ Sleep anxiety

■ Risk Factors

The ones that make you more prone to developing insomnia include:

+ A family history of insomnia.
+ A history of sleep troubles in the past.
+ Getting older.
+ Being female.
+ Having anxiety or depression.
+ A history of trauma.
+ Having health anxiety.
+ Having high sensitivity to feeling bad after getting little sleep.
+ Having a perfectionistic or Type A personality.
+ Having a strong desire for control in your life.

■ Triggering Event Leads to Initial Sleep Disruption

Next, there is a **triggering event** that brings on an *initial episode* of sleep disruption. This is almost always stress-related.

For example, people might have a period of poor sleep when they have:

+ Intense pressure at work.
+ A major loss such as the death of a family member.

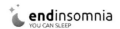

+ Stressful relationships or interpersonal issues.

+ A new baby.

+ Financial worries.

+ A health scare.

This short-term sleep disruption can also result from certain drugs and medications, high levels of stimulation right before bed—and even from being really excited about something.

Occasional short-term sleep disruption is normal and unavoidable. It happens to everyone.

Usually, sleep returns to normal when the stressor passes or when a person adjusts to the change.

What Turns Short-Term Sleep Issues Into Long-Term Insomnia?

But sometimes, short-term insomnia becomes long-term insomnia. Why? It comes down to anxiety.

Anxiety about sleeplessness and its daytime consequences is the root cause of the problem.

When you can't sleep and it feels distressing, and you have to suffer the next-day consequences, it's easy to get anxious about how you'll sleep the next night and how you'll sleep in the long-term future.

Because of the body-mind connection, when you are anxious about sleep and feel threatened by the prospect of not sleeping, it triggers nervous system **hyperarousal.**

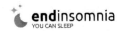

Hyperarousal is a state of nervous system activation that occurs when you are stressed or are under threat. When you experience hyperarousal, your nervous system enters into a fight-or-flight state in which your body readies itself to fend off or escape from danger.

In this state, your body releases stress hormones, your heart rate may increase, muscle tension increases, and your brain becomes more active.

This nervous system response happens automatically to help you respond to the perception of danger. Your conscious will is not involved. If you were to encounter a threat like a wild predatory animal, entering into a state of hyperarousal in this automatic way would help you run, fight, or otherwise survive.

Although hyperarousal is a nervous system response aimed at survival, you can go into hyperarousal even when you're not in physical danger. For example, you might experience hyperarousal when you are dealing with general life stressors or if you are simply anxious about the possibility of not sleeping.

At night, hyperarousal can cause you to:

+ Experience "hypnic jerks," or involuntary jerks in your body that jolt you awake just as you're falling asleep (sometimes accompanied by a feeling of falling).

+ Wake up in an anxious and activated state during the night, making it hard to re-enter sleep.

+ Experience an accelerated heart rate as you lie in bed, feeling increasingly anxious about how you will sleep.

+ Overly monitor the process of falling asleep.

+ Drift in and out of light sleep for much of the night.

+ Be tense and on edge and feel like sleep is very far away, even if you are exhausted.

So anxiety and the accompanying hyperarousal make it very hard to sleep.

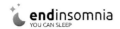

When someone has insomnia (which often feels like a problem nobody else has) and experiences all kinds of distress at night, it's easy for them to believe that "something is wrong with" them.

Let me reassure you that you are not broken. Insomnia is not a condition the way heart disease or cancer is a condition. Its root is ultimately not in the body but in the mind. The fundamental issue is anxiety and the nervous system activation that follows from anxiety.

While insomnia ultimately has a psychological root, I'm not saying it's your fault. On the contrary, insomnia starts due to a perfect storm of factors, many of which are outside your control. Once it gets established, it's challenging to break free from.

Recognizing that insomnia has a psychological root doesn't mean the suffering you experience isn't "real." It just means there is a way out.

You can bring an end to your sleep issues by undergoing a psychological transformation (which also has the effect of reversing your nervous system hyperarousal) using the system laid out in Part 2 of this book.

Sleep Anxiety and the Factors That Drive Ongoing Insomnia

Sleep anxiety and the nervous system hyperarousal that accompanies it make it difficult to sleep, even when you're really tired. As a response to the distress of not sleeping, especially as sleep problems carry on over time, people with insomnia generally take up the following "Unhelpfuls" that end up feeding and maintaining sleep anxiety:

+ **Unhelpful perceptions**
+ **Unhelpful reactions**
+ **Unhelpful behaviors**

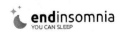

I'll explain each in more detail—but the upshot is that each of these "Unhelpfuls" reinforce each other and amplify your sleep issues.

Let's break these factors down.

■ Unhelpful Perceptions

Perceptions that drive your sleep anxiety and hyperarousal include your understanding of what's happening, your thoughts about your experience, and your mindset about it.

Some examples of perceptions that fuel insomnia include:

+ Misunderstandings about why you are sleeping badly and what that means about you.

+ Misinformation about what normal sleep is.

+ Extreme evaluations of how bad your situation is and how bad your future might be as a result.

When you are misinformed about insomnia and how sleep works, it's easy to assume the worst and create an inaccurate story about what's happening that makes you even more anxious.

You can change the unhelpful and inaccurate perceptions that drive insomnia by gaining knowledge that shifts your understanding. This whole book is full of knowledge aimed at changing unhelpful perceptions.

Additionally, your perceptions will change by having new experiences that lead to greater confidence in your ability to sleep and handle the challenges of insomnia with less suffering. I offer ways to change your perceptions about insomnia throughout the book—and you'll also be guided to make some explicit shifts in thinking in Part 2.

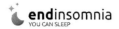

■ Unhelpful Reactions

The reactions that fuel sleep anxiety and hyperarousal include:

+ Emotional volatility when you don't sleep well or when you experience daytime fatigue.

+ Struggling against difficult emotions or the presence of uncertainty.

+ Fixating on your sleep difficulties.

+ Trying to force sleep to happen.

+ Berating yourself when you are struggling.

+ Giving up when the going gets tough.

In Part 2, you will learn how to be less reactive to your insomnia in these unhelpful ways. You will do this by becoming more informed about your situation and through learning mindful acceptance, strategies to manage difficult thoughts and feelings, and self-compassion.

■ Unhelpful Behaviors

Behaviors that drive sleep anxiety and hyperarousal (and beyond that, would make it hard to sleep even if you felt calm) are any actions you take that undermine your body's natural ability to feel tired and fall asleep. These include spending far too long in bed and taking long naps during the day.

Trying to force yourself to sleep through willpower, and making major sacrifices in your life to try to get your insomnia under control, also fall under the category of unhelpful behaviors.

This book will guide you to correct any unhelpful behaviors you might have and adopt a new set of sleep-supporting habits.

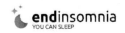
When Hyperarousal Becomes Conditioned

Long-term insomnia is driven by a vicious cycle. Sleep anxiety and the associated hyperarousal make it hard to sleep. In turn, the distress of not sleeping and the consequences lead to perceptions of threat, high reactivity to challenging situations, and sleep-undermining behaviors feed your anxiety and make it even harder to sleep. Increased sleep anxiety and sleep troubles then lead to more unhelpful responses, and so on.

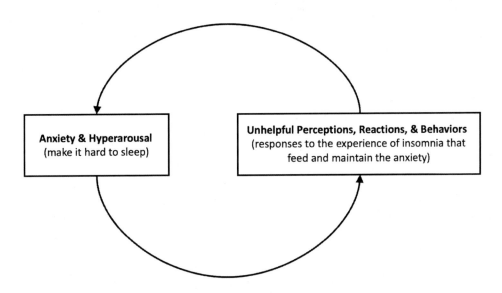

Anxiety & Hyperarousal
(make it hard to sleep)

Unhelpful Perceptions, Reactions, & Behaviors
(responses to the experience of insomnia that feed and maintain the anxiety)

As the vicious cycle of insomnia continues and you have many nights of bad sleep, and you experience a lot of anxiety and dread about your sleep, your body can become **conditioned** to automatically enter into a state of hyperarousal ("**conditioned hyperarousal**") as bedtime approaches, as you climb into bed, or throughout the whole night. This means that even if you're not consciously feeling too anxious about your sleep, your nervous system can enter into a fight-or-flight state on its own, based on learned associations and past conditioning.

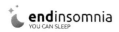

This can help explain why you might feel very sleepy a few minutes before heading to bed but then suddenly feel agitated and wide awake once you get into bed. This explains why you might wake up from sleep in the middle of the night and notice your body is in a state of alarm (even if you hadn't been consciously feeling anxious—you were just asleep).

The experience of conditioned hyperarousal is enormously frustrating for someone with insomnia. Not only are you already anxious and distressed about your sleep, but your body has learned to enter a state of hyperarousal on its own. You desperately want your body to be calm so you can sleep, but your body has been conditioned to experience the night as a dangerous and threatening time, which makes it even harder to sleep. **Unfortunately, your body's automatic threat system is not sophisticated enough to realize that its vigilance is backfiring.**

Your nervous system activates in response to the threat of not sleeping, which is the very thing that prevents you from sleeping, which triggers an even deeper sense of threat. Even if your conscious mind knows it's safe to sleep, your subconscious mind and your nervous system have been conditioned to believe it's not.

You may be getting the sense that this situation is a job for something more than herbal tea! Or sleeping pills, relaxation techniques, or sleep hygiene protocols.

You're right: When your body reacts as if you are in life-threatening danger, these flimsy interventions don't stand a chance.

While these things sometimes can help short-term—possibly due to the "placebo effect"—you need **long-term strategies** to **calm the anxiety at the root** of insomnia.

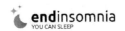

Reversing the Factors That Maintain Insomnia

We want to get you to a point where you're sleeping well every night. To get there, *you need to target the sleep anxiety at the root of it all.* This will involve working to **reverse** the unhelpful perceptions, reactions, and behaviors that keep the vicious cycle of insomnia going.

As you do so, the conditioned hyperarousal will lessen over time until it's no longer a problem.

The diagram below shows the process of reversing your insomnia.

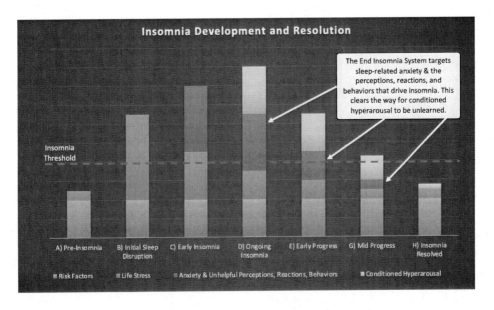

In bar B of the graph shown, high stress levels after some challenging life event trigger initial sleep disruption, bringing you above the insomnia threshold. In bar C, sleep anxiety and accompanying unhelpful perceptions, reactions, and behaviors develop.

Insomnia takes on a life of its own even after the initial stressor fades away or you adjust to it. In bar D, ongoing insomnia leads to conditioned hyperarousal, making your insomnia even worse.

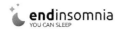

Bars D, E, and G show how the End Insomnia System targets your sleep anxiety, along with the perceptions, reactions, and behaviors that keep the vicious cycle going. As your sleep anxiety is lowered over time, the conditioned hyperarousal decreases naturally.

One encouraging fact is that whenever you work with one of these areas—unhelpful perceptions, reactions, or behaviors—the other two are also positively affected.

For example, if you learn more about what's going on with your sleep and correct faulty perceptions, you will become less afraid.

When you're less afraid, you will be less reactive.

When you are less reactive, you become less prone to unhelpful behaviors.

If you work to become less reactive to your distress and sleep issues, you will build a perception that the situation is less threatening, and it will be easier to stick to sleep-promoting behaviors.

If you make behavioral changes to support long-term good sleep and see some positive change, your perceptions of fear and threat will ease as you gain more confidence—and it will also be easier to be less reactive because you will be less afraid. So there are many different ways to help yourself.

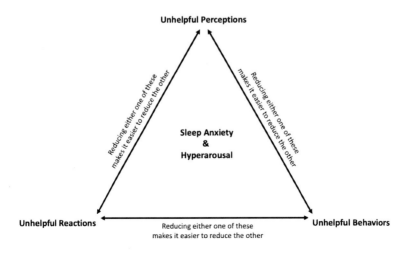

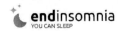

Additionally, taking steps to be less anxious at night makes for easier days. Why? Because when you're calm at night, not only do you have a higher chance of falling asleep, but you'll feel more calm and rested the next day even if you don't sleep great. In a similar way, taking steps to ease your suffering during the day makes it easier to sleep at night because you'll be less anxious about the daytime consequences of not sleeping.

So interventions *at any of the problem points* affect the whole.

Piece by piece, you will become less anxious about the situation and move closer to full resolution of your insomnia.

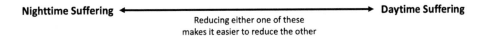

In the next few chapters, you'll learn that you have *limited control* over how you sleep on a *night-to-night* basis.

However, you have *a lot of control* over sleeping well in the *long term*.

Part 2 will give you a framework for creating long-term changes to achieve great sleep while working to lessen your anxiety about how you sleep in the short term.

You'll learn how to truly care less about how you sleep on any given night and to build a sense of healthy non-attachment to how you sleep that will help your nervous system be much more sleep-compatible at night.

You don't need to become completely unafraid and completely unattached in order to overcome your insomnia. You just need to get to a point where there is no longer a deep sense of menace regarding your sleep. When you follow the steps of the End Insomnia System and reduce your anxiety enough, your sleep will start to improve, and with time your hyperarousal will settle.

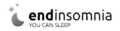

Where You Are Headed

When all of this is done, you will be sleeping well consistently—and even if you occasionally experience a bad night, it won't be such a big deal. Due to the work you have done to reduce your sleep anxiety, you will have strong protection against spiraling into insomnia in the future. You will be free to focus on living the life you want to live.

At the end of your journey of overcoming insomnia, you will have gained a powerful set of skills for working with your thoughts and emotions and for dealing more effectively with all kinds of difficulties that you may encounter in your life.

Although it may sound hard to believe, some who use this approach, once they reach the end phases of the healing process, say that if they could go back in time and choose whether or not to have insomnia, they would choose to have insomnia again.

This is not because this system turns them into masochists. Rather, their journey through insomnia left them no choice but to learn how to find calmness and even-mindedness in the face of enormous difficulty. As a result, they are now much better at handling stress, they feel empowered and proud of themselves, and they have learned how to meet the challenges of life with greater acceptance, flexibility, compassion, and perspective.

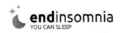

SELF-ASSESSMENT:
WHERE YOU STAND TO GROW

This self-assessment will show you where you stand to grow as you apply the End Insomnia System to the anxiety underlying your sleep issues. Don't worry if your score is low—the point is to give you a sense of the sorts of experiences you will have as you learn to apply the End Insomnia System.

Below, rate yourself on a scale from 0–4 on how accurate the statements are; 0 means "not true for me at all," and 4 means "very true for me."

Once you've filled a rating for each statement, total up your numbers and use the scoring system below the self-assessment.

OVERCOMING INSOMNIA CHECK-IN STATEMENT	SELF RATING
1. I have a clear sense of why I have insomnia and the steps that I can take to overcome it in a lasting and sustainable way.	
2. I am confident that I can handle my thoughts without feeling trapped in them and without getting stuck in rumination (being totally caught up in repetitive thoughts).	
3. The presence of worrisome thoughts doesn't cause me to spiral into panic, and I don't automatically believe my thoughts as objective truth.	

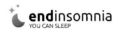
OVERCOMING INSOMNIA CHECK-IN STATEMENT	SELF RATING

4. I am confident in my ability to manage difficult emotions with acceptance and tolerance while also not getting completely lost in them.

5. I feel relatively calm and patient at night when I can't sleep, and I don't try to force it.

6. When my body has hyperarousal symptoms, I understand what's going on and remain calm without reacting in unhelpful ways.

7. I am confident that the amount of time I choose to spend in bed each night is helping my sleep, and sticking to this time window doesn't cause me much anxiety even when I'm having poor sleep.

8. I no longer do things like keep an exact and fine-tuned wind-down routine, follow rigid rules or rituals before bed to increase my chances of sleep, or organize my day around trying to increase my chances of getting sleep that night. Instead, my behaviors are pretty much like they were before I had insomnia.

9. I don't blame myself when I can't sleep or when my body experiences hyperarousal. Instead, I generally treat myself with kindness and understanding when I'm struggling.

10. I have come to see that the most difficult nights and fatigued days are actually valuable opportunities for me to keep working through insomnia if I respond in appropriate ways.

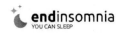

OVERCOMING INSOMNIA CHECK-IN STATEMENT	SELF RATING
11. I remain confident in my path to better sleep even when I have a bad night.	
12. When I experience poor sleep after a period of good sleep, I understand what's happening. I know how to respond, get back on track quickly, and have my sleep confidence actually benefit from the setback.	
13. I feel increasingly indifferent to or unattached to how I sleep on a night-to-night basis, and I know I am continually working toward lasting great sleep in the long term.	
14. I feel confident that I can get through my day and do things that give me meaning and fulfillment, even when I'm faced with fatigue or difficult emotions.	
15. I sometimes feel grateful for my insomnia. (This one doesn't tend to happen until you start seeing the light on the other side.) The experience has helped me to learn about my mind, to relate to my thoughts and emotions in much more intentional and effective ways, and it has given me more empathy for others experiencing difficulties in life.	
16. I don't feel triggered when I have a thought about insomnia or if I hear "sleep" or "insomnia" brought up during the day.	

TOTAL UP YOUR SCORE:

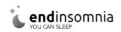

What Your Score Means

Score: 0–25
Ready for Change

You are ready for change. You've been through a lot, and the way out of this mess is not yet clear. The thoughts, feelings, hyperarousal, and unwanted wakefulness that accompany insomnia may often feel more than you can bear.

The End Insomnia System will give you a path to reach all of the experiences listed in the self-assessment above. You are ripe for transformation. Read on.

Score: 26–50
Finding Your Way

You've likely been exposed to some helpful sources of information about insomnia and have managed to cultivate some resilience to poor sleep. You have likely developed some resilience in the face of the difficult thoughts, feelings, and circumstances you encounter with insomnia.

The End Insomnia System will take your progress and build upon it. We'll fill in the gaps in your knowledge and address the points where you still struggle with specific practices and perspectives that can move you closer to fully living out the types of experiences listed in the self-assessment statements.

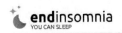

Score: 50–64
Mastery Over Insomnia

Nice! If you score in this range, you're in a great position. You've done a lot of work to reverse the anxiety that drives insomnia and have found ways to relate to challenging thoughts, feelings, and circumstances with greater acceptance, self-compassion, and flexibility.

If you are not completely past your insomnia yet, you are well on your way. If you find yourself with this score on your first read-through of the book, then you will likely find that the End Insomnia System can build upon the great progress you've already made.

This system will provide you with knowledge, perspective, and practices you may not have yet considered that can guide you through the final stretch of your journey to consistent great sleep.

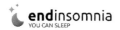

GET EXTRA HELP

Do you want to get to a life free from insomnia as quickly and painlessly as possible? Our **End Insomnia Program** will help you do just that. If you join, you'll get:

+ An engaging video course that drives home everything you'll learn in this book.

+ Tools to help you apply what you're learning in a structured way.

+ Accountability to help you keep on track—and encourage you when you're struggling.

+ Group coaching calls to get ongoing live support and do deeper dives into the topics in the book. Wherever you are in the process of working through insomnia, the calls provide guidance and help to take you to the next level. We also deconstruct individual stories and situations, so everyone can learn from them.

+ A supportive community of others working through insomnia. The community provides support, encouragement, and empathy. You can find peers to lean on and get help and advice from others on the journey. You can also get your questions answered by coaches on the community platform.

CHECK IT OUT:

https://endinsomnia.com/program

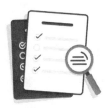

KEY CHAPTER TAKEAWAYS

☑ Insomnia develops in a predictable way. It is fueled by sleep anxiety and hyperarousal; unhelpful perceptions, reactions, behaviors; and conditioning.

☑ As you reverse the unhelpful perceptions, reactions, and behaviors, your sleep anxiety will lessen, as will the conditioned hyperarousal that seems to make your body go haywire at night.

☑ Once you learn to care less about how you sleep, you will no longer experience the perception of threat at night that gets in the way of sleep.

CHAPTER

4

The Sleep-Starting Force and the Sleep-Stopping Force

In the last chapter, we went over the science of sleep. In this chapter, I'm going to make it even more simple.

Sleep is controlled by only two things: I call them the **sleep-starting force** and the **sleep-stopping force.**

The Sleep-Starting Force

First, let's talk about what I call the **sleep-starting force**. This is what induces sleep. It consists of two biological systems in your body. These are your *sleep drive* and *circadian rhythm*.

Your *sleep drive* is the biological pressure to sleep that builds each hour you're awake and active. The only way to lower your ever-growing sleep drive is to sleep. Sleep is a core biological need that must be met. Your sleep drive will not allow you to go too long without sleep. Eventually, your sleep drive will force you to sleep.

Your *circadian rhythm* is the internal body clock that makes you feel sleepy and awake at predictable times. This inner clock allows your body to trigger

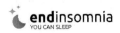

wakefulness and sleepiness based on your past sleep schedule and cues such as daylight that keep the cycle of biological processes in your body consistent.

Your sleep drive and circadian rhythm work together to manage wakefulness and sleepiness. You have a lower sleep drive when you wake up in the morning because you just slept. As your sleep drive builds during the day, you may feel tired in the afternoon. Then the circadian rhythm gives you another kick of wakefulness until the evening when your sleep drive and circadian rhythm synchronize to create a high level of sleepiness around bedtime.

Here's an example of the sleep drive and circadian rhythm working together for a typical adult:

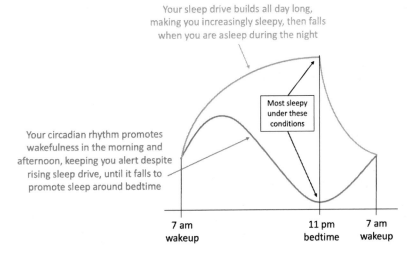

The sleep drive and circadian rhythm that make up the sleep-starting force are the *only things that can induce sleep.*

Nothing outside of these two biological systems can do this.

That is good news because it means you are not responsible for "making" sleep happen. Sleep is a passive biological process that occurs on its own. Your body does it automatically for you. Normal sleepers don't need to do anything to make themselves sleep because the sleep-starting force simply takes over without any effort on their part.

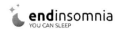

The biological sleep-starting force cannot be broken. It's always there waiting to help you sleep, and it will help you do so much more easily once you lower the sleep-stopping force.

The Sleep-Stopping Force

If the sleep-starting force is supposed to make you sleep automatically without any effort, why do you have so much trouble sleeping? The sleep-stopping force is responsible for your troubles.

What I call the sleep-stopping force is the anxiety and hyperarousal that keep your body wired—and awake—even when the biological conditions for sleep are otherwise present.

When you are experiencing a great deal of stress and anxiety, your brain responds by turning on the fight-or-flight nervous system response, which is intended to help you survive threatening situations. For example, if you encountered a bear in the woods, your body would automatically go into fight-or-flight mode. Your body primes itself to run for your life or fight the bear. There is a good reason for this: your brain is aware of the presence of a threat and doesn't want you to die.

Do you know what would be hard? Lying down and going to sleep while the bear stood over you.

Lying down with insomnia is the same challenge.

The perception of threat and the accompanying nervous system response is the basis of the sleep-stopping force. When your body's fight-or-flight threat response is activated, your ability to sleep is temporarily inhibited. To the more primal part of your brain, it is more important to be alert when a threat is present than to sleep, even if your body is quite fatigued.

With insomnia, the threat keeping you awake is the prospect of not sleeping.

Unfortunately, your nervous system is not sophisticated enough to understand that the fight-or-flight response triggered by the threat of not sleeping is the

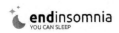

very thing that prevents you from sleeping. In this way, you can get stuck in a looping threat response. Your anxiety about not sleeping creates a nervous system response that makes it hard to sleep, which leads to an even greater sense of threat that makes it *even harder* to sleep, which... and so on.

While this can seem like a bleak situation, you'll see the way out in the chapters to come.

High Sleep-Starting Force + Low Sleep-Stopping Force = Effortless Sleep

In the diagram shown here, you can see the relationship between the sleep-starting force, the sleep-stopping force, and your ability to sleep.

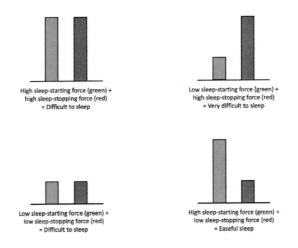

Various Scenarios of The Sleep-Starting Force (Green) vs. Sleep-Stopping Force (Red)

High sleep-starting force (green) +
high sleep-stopping force (red)
= Difficult to sleep

Low sleep-starting force (green) +
high sleep-stopping force (red)
= Very difficult to sleep

Low sleep-starting force (green) +
low sleep-stopping force (red)
= Difficult to sleep

High sleep-starting force (green) +
low sleep-stopping force (red)
= Easeful sleep

When both the sleep-starting force and sleep-stopping force are high, your body is ready to sleep, but a high level of nervous system arousal gets in the way and makes it difficult to sleep. If you stay in this state long enough or accumulate multiple nights of poor sleep, you will eventually sleep. The sleep-starting force will eventually grow strong enough to overpower any anxiety and nervous system arousal that you might have.

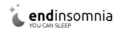

When the sleep-starting force is low and the sleep-stopping force is high, your body is not ready for sleep, and your nervous system is not in a sleep-compatible state. This combination will make it nearly impossible to fall asleep.

When the sleep-starting force and sleep-stopping force are both low, you're not very anxious or on edge, but your body's need for sleep is also not high, so it will be difficult to sleep.

The ideal state is to have a high sleep-starting force and a low sleep-stopping force. This combination makes for effortless sleep.

The End Insomnia System draws on a range of strategies to dial up your sleep-starting force in a gentle and sustainable way (you'll learn how in Chapter 8) and dial *down* your sleep-stopping force (covered in Chapters 9–15).

When you do these two things, sleep happens—without effort. And you will begin to gain confidence in your natural ability to sleep.

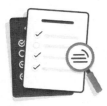

KEY CHAPTER TAKEAWAYS

☑   The only thing that makes you sleep is the **sleep-starting force** (your sleep drive plus your *circadian rhythm*).

☑   The **sleep-stopping force** (*anxiety and hyperarousal*) is what gets in the way of sleep.

☑   To address insomnia, you need to *increase* the sleep-starting force while decreasing the sleep-stopping force.

CHAPTER 5

Sleep Efforts

This chapter will examine why many of the ways you've tried to address your insomnia have failed—including sleeping pills, nighttime rituals, relaxation exercises, and more. **You will also take your first actions to begin addressing your insomnia in a better way.** Let's jump in.

When you are highly anxious at night, full of hyperarousal, and dreading how you will feel tomorrow if you don't sleep soon, the most natural response is to try to do something to make yourself sleep. Often when we encounter a painful or stressful situation in life, the first thing we do is engage in problem-solving. This strategy works well for many situations, but it doesn't work for solving the problem of not being able to sleep.

The reason problem-solving strategies aimed at making you sleep don't work is that sleep is a passive biological process. You can't turn on sleep using your willpower.

Just as you don't have conscious control over your digestion or the beating of your heart, you don't have control over the process of falling and staying asleep. As mentioned in the last chapter, the only things that control your ability to fall and stay asleep are the **sleep-starting force** (sleep drive and circadian rhythm) and the **sleep-stopping force** (anxiety and hyperarousal).

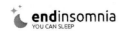

What Are Sleep Efforts and Why Are They a Problem?

We'll use the term "sleep efforts" to refer to the various ways you may have tried to force sleep to happen. Sleep efforts are one of the most common "unhelpful behaviors" referenced in the last chapter—doing something is usually the first place our minds go when we can't sleep.

Sleep efforts include anything aimed at trying to force sleep to happen in the night ahead, such as:

+ Elaborate pre-bedtime rituals.

+ Using relaxation exercises as you lie in bed awake to try to induce sleep.

+ Micromanaging your sleep environment.

+ Taking sleeping pills.

+ Anything else you do or avoid in your life in order to try to get control over how you sleep tonight.

Unfortunately, apart from sleep efforts not working, engaging in them actually makes you *less likely* to fall asleep. There are two reasons for this.

First, when you regard being awake at night as a high-stakes problem that you must fix through effort, you reinforce the message to your mind and body that you are under threat. When your mind perceives that you are under threat, you don't sleep. Normal sleepers don't make sleep efforts and don't feel under threat at night. They just get into bed and sleep eventually happens. The End Insomnia System will get you to that way of experiencing sleep.

Second, because sleep efforts don't work, you will often feel additionally frustrated, anxious, and desperate when you try to force yourself to sleep and then fail. More emotional distress means more nervous system arousal, making it harder to sleep..

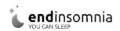

To show you what I mean, let's try an experiment:

1. Take this book with you.

2. Go lie down. (Yes, now, if possible. If not, try this tonight in bed.)

3. Lying down? Good. Now:

4. Close your eyes, and

5. SLEEP! NOW!

How'd that go?

Even a normal sleeper can't will themselves to sleep. It's folly to think someone with insomnia could.

So even though sleep efforts can seem like the best option in the moment, they actually make the problem worse and should be stopped.

However, *stopping sleep efforts is just the first step* to ending your insomnia. At this point, even if you stop all your sleep efforts, you are still going to have a lot of trouble sleeping—because your *sleep-stopping force* is still high.

The End Insomnia System has a solution for this: *gradually decrease* your sleep-stopping force—while *increasing* your sleep-starting force at night.

You'll learn how in Part 2.

Let's now take a deeper dive into common sleep efforts. Keep an eye out for any that apply to you. We'll look separately at nighttime sleep efforts and daytime sleep efforts.

This section will also explain why many of the "solutions" you've used to try to sleep better have not actually fixed your problem.

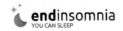

Sleep Efforts at Night

■ Spending Too Much Time in Bed Trying to Sleep

One unhelpful (but tempting) way to try to get more control over your sleep is to spend extra hours in bed. For example, you might try to scrape together some extra sleep by going to bed an hour early or staying in bed after you would normally get up. Spending too long in bed at night sabotages your sleep drive for the next night and interferes with your long-term ability to overcome insomnia.

We'll discuss how long to spend in bed in Chapter 8.

■ Medications or Other Substances

Another common way people with insomnia try to make themselves sleep at night is by taking prescription sleeping pills or other substances such as alcohol or cannabis. While many medical providers are quick to prescribe sleeping pills for insomnia, there are three reasons these are not good solutions for insomnia.

First, many pills and substances have side effects that can leave you feeling groggy or worse the next day. One side effect of alcohol, THC, and sleeping pills is that they can interfere with the natural processes that occur in various sleep stages that help you feel restored.

Even if such "sleep aids" do help you get a little more sleep, you may feel unrested when you wake up after using them. Many report they feel worse after getting sleeping pill–assisted sleep than they do when they get less sleep without sleeping pills.

Second, the effectiveness of using these sorts of sleep aids tends to drop off over time. One reason is that your body builds up tolerance, so over time, higher doses are needed to have the same effect.

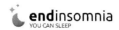

The other reason for a drop in effectiveness is that the initial boost of confidence and hope a new pill or substance gives you (the "placebo effect") can't stand up to chronic sleep anxiety in the long term. You begin to doubt your sleep aids when they don't work as well as they did at first, and so they lose the ability to make you feel as calm psychologically. In this way, the placebo effect of taking the pill or substance wears off over time.

Third, taking pills, or substances to try to make yourself sleep undermines your faith in your natural ability to sleep. This point can't be overstated. As long as you are taking a sleeping aid, you can't fully come to believe that sleep will happen without it. Your pills and substances become a physical symbol of the fear you have about not sleeping and a reminder of how attached you are to your sleep going a certain way.

For these reasons, there comes a time in your insomnia journey when it's important to let these substances go—and face your sleep anxiety so you can overcome it.

Some may begin to let go of their pills, or substances immediately. Others may choose to let them go at some point down the line, which is also okay.

As you learn the tools and perspectives in this book, they will give you a new anchor to hold onto that will provide a sense of confidence and greater safety. Once you are firmly holding this new anchor, it is much easier to let go of the old one.

If you choose to come off sleeping pills as you work with the system provided in this book, *do not go off them cold turkey.* Doing so can result in a physical withdrawal that can cause a spike in your insomnia symptoms and cause you unnecessary suffering. *It's critical to work with your medical provider to safely wean yourself off prescription sleeping pills once you choose to do so.*

If you are tapering off non-prescription sleeping medication, you might try a quarter-dose to half-dose reduction every two weeks.

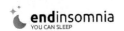

■ Relaxation and Imagination Exercises

At night, when you can't sleep, you might have tried various techniques to induce sleep, such as breathing techniques, relaxation exercises, meditation, or imagining a vivid scene. If you use any of these with the *intention* to force sleep to happen, they won't work.

For someone with a normal low-stakes relationship with sleep, these kinds of strategies may help soothe their nervous system and help them drift off. This is not true for people with insomnia because they don't have a normal relationship with sleep.

These techniques are not powerful enough to settle the sense of threat that people with insomnia experience. Instead, making these efforts just reinforces the notion that something threatening is happening.

■ Desperately Trying to Control Your Thoughts

You might have also blamed your inability to sleep on the presence of anxious thoughts and desperately tried to fight them off. You might also have employed a technique called "thought challenging".

It can absolutely be helpful to challenge anxiety-fueling thoughts that may not be realistic. We will describe the healthy way to do so in Chapter 10. However, if you approach thought challenging with an inflexible and desperate intention— believing that you must make these thoughts go away or else your night will be ruined—the stakes may be too high for thought challenging to help calm you down. Ultimately, it takes more than some thought challenging to shift the level of anxiety you have around not sleeping, which is why the End Insomnia System exists.

If you believe you cannot sleep until anxious thoughts leave you, Chapters 9 and 10 will show you helpful ways to relate to those thoughts so you can learn that they don't need to be totally gone for you to sleep. Also, in Chapter 11, you will learn about realistic attitudes to adopt toward sleep, which will naturally help your thoughts become more reasonable and less extreme.

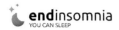
Daytime and Pre-Bedtime Sleep Efforts

There are also a number of sleep efforts you might be making during the day or in the hours leading up to bedtime aimed at controlling your sleep that night.

■ Rituals Before Bed

Out of desperation, people with insomnia often do all kinds of rituals leading up to bed to try to increase their chances of sleep. For example, you may have tried having a carefully timed bath to drop your body temperature in hopes of inducing sleep. Or perhaps you have an evening cup of herbal tea, smell lavender essential oil, or use relaxation techniques for a certain amount of time before you go to bed.

Apart from being sleep efforts—which don't work—all these sorts of rituals end up holding you back because they undermine your faith in your natural ability to sleep without effort. It's hard to have confidence that you can sleep under flexible conditions (like a normal sleeper does) when you feel like you must do an hour's worth of rituals to possibly have a chance at sleep. That's not the relationship we want you to have with sleep going forward.

■ Exercise

In a bid for sleep, you may have tried to tire yourself out physically during the day through exercise. Exercise is great for mental and physical health; it's worth doing and may even help you sleep a little more deeply. However, if you exercise with the sole intention of wearing yourself out in hopes that you sleep better, then that's a sleep effort and will likely backfire.

Additionally, when you spend a lot of time making daytime sleep efforts (like exercising), you may create even more performance anxiety about sleep because you are anxious to see whether or not those efforts will come through for you.

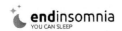

■ Avoiding Blue Light

There's truth to the idea that avoiding blue light (emitted by screens) before bed can help support sleep, but someone with insomnia might develop extreme beliefs about how critical following this rule is.

Substantial blue light exposure at night can delay your circadian rhythm a bit because it can signal to your body that it is day, rather than night. This could slightly interfere with your sleep-starting force. However, many normal sleepers look at screens before bed and sleep completely fine. If you have insomnia and you hear about this rule, you might stop looking at screens several hours before bed and feel quite uneasy being around screens or lights in the evening.

Let's take a look at some research. A much-cited study from 2014 examined the effect on sleep of using an iPad for several hours before bed. The study found that extended blue light exposure before bed did suppress melatonin production and cause a delay in the circadian rhythm.

However, in the study, the people who looked at an iPad for 4 hours straight before bed *took only 10 minutes longer* to get to sleep than people who read a book in the hours before bed. This is not a huge effect.

While it's generally a good idea to avoid staring at screens close to bedtime for the reasons mentioned, don't worry about following this rule militantly. The root cause of your trouble sleeping is anxiety and hyperarousal, not blue light. If you do end up using screens close to bedtime, try to avoid highly stimulating content, such as upsetting news, social media, or intense movies.

■ Micromanaging Bedroom Conditions

You might have also tried to get control over the process of falling asleep by trying to change your bedroom into a place with perfect quiet, total darkness, or an exact room temperature. While it's generally sleep-conducive to be in a reasonably quiet, dark, and cool environment, if you feel you cannot possibly sleep without your bedroom conditions being exactly right, you are being ruled by sleep anxiety.

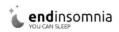

Work on challenging the belief that your sleep conditions must be perfect for you to sleep. The sleep-stopping force (sleep anxiety and hyperarousal) is the real issue, not your bedroom conditions.

■ Withdrawing From Your Life to Get Control Over Your Sleep

Finally, a primary way people try to take control of their sleep in the short term and end up sabotaging themselves in the long term is by withdrawing from their lives to try to sleep better.

When you have insomnia and it feels out of control, it's easy to start giving up on activities that are important to you. You may give things up to try to increase your chances of sleeping, or perhaps simply because you feel like you cannot handle them anymore due to your fatigue and anxiety.

Unfortunately, the more you sacrifice parts of your life to manage your insomnia, the more insomnia becomes the center of your life and the more anxious you will become about it.

Due to insomnia, you might cut back on work or school, withdraw from your social life, cut back on hobbies, stop drinking all caffeine, or make any number of other adjustments to make your life smaller. These are understandable responses if you feel at the end of your rope and miserable. The idea of living with gusto and ambition when you have insomnia doesn't seem to make much sense.

But guess what? The situation starts to change as you gain faith that there is a path to permanently overcome insomnia, and you begin to walk that path with persistence. As your confidence builds in the process, there comes a time when you must begin to re-engage more fully with your life, even if it feels hard at first.

It will feel challenging for a while, but living more fully is a key element in becoming less afraid and less attached to how you sleep each night. Life will then become easier as you work through your insomnia and your sleep begins to improve. We'll talk about a framework for engaging fully in your life in greater detail in Chapter 12.

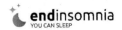
Letting Go of Sleep Efforts Effectively

You have likely had times when it seemed like your sleep efforts helped you sleep. It's easy to hold onto those memories and try those sleep efforts again when you get desperate. It's important to remember that you truly cannot force yourself to sleep. The only things that control sleep are the sleep-starting force (sleep drive and circadian rhythm) and the sleep-stopping force (anxiety and hyperarousal). That's it.

So, how can we understand times when it seemed like your sleep efforts helped? They certainly didn't induce sleep because they don't have any impact on the sleep-starting force. So they would've had to have had some kind of impact on the sleep-stopping force.

It is true that certain sleep efforts can temporarily reduce the anxiety that keeps you awake, but they do so in an unsustainable and ultimately unhelpful way.

There are a couple of reasons why sleep efforts sometimes seem to help. First, there's the "placebo effect" — when you believe something will help you sleep, it can give you a temporary boost of confidence and hope. For example, when you do a certain ritual before bed, it might give you a sense of relief because you believe it increases your likelihood of sleeping.

However, the reality is that such efforts do not help you sleep and actually work against you by turning sleep into a performance. In this way, many sleep efforts that have seemed to work in the past are just psychological crutches that give you a little bit of false ease but ultimately stand in the way of attaining normal sleep.

Similar logic applies to why pills can seem to help a little bit. Pills and sedating substances can have a dampening effect on your nervous system arousal. However, it's important to recognize that these pills aren't inducing sleep. They're just temporarily dampening the nervous system arousal that interferes with sleep. And as mentioned previously, pills and substances have many drawbacks and ultimately get in the way of truly addressing your insomnia.

To overcome insomnia, you need to get to the heart of your sleep anxiety and overcome it in a way that following rituals or taking a pill will never allow you to do.

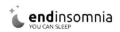

The End Insomnia System is designed to do precisely that. We don't try to put a band-aid over your sleep anxiety or just block it out so you can sleep better for one night. No, this is a system that, over time, will uproot your sleep anxiety so that it is truly not there anymore.

However, to be in a position where that's possible, you need to give up sleep efforts that don't serve you and that keep you stuck in dysfunctional beliefs about how sleep works and what you need to do to sleep.

If you find yourself reverting to old sleep efforts in a moment of desperation, know that is a normal part of the process. Just recognize that you're engaging in a sleep effort—and get back on track. Don't beat yourself up or feel that you've majorly set back your progress. As long as you get back on track quickly—and don't compound your stress by berating yourself for having engaged in a sleep effort—it is not a big deal.

GET HELP ENDING YOUR SLEEP EFFORTS

Sleep efforts can be subtle and automatic. Even when you think you've given them up, they can sneak back into your habits without you realizing it.

To get help sorting out your sleep efforts and to receive support and expert knowledge when you slip up or feel stuck, join the **End Insomnia Program**. It's the best way to apply everything you learn in this book to see results as fast as possible.

Our coaches, course, and community are invaluable companions as you work to overcome your insomnia. We'll help you up when you're down and guide you through any points of confusion you encounter.

LEARN MORE HERE:

https://endinsomnia.com/program

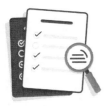

KEY CHAPTER TAKEAWAYS

☑ **Sleep efforts** are anything you do in the day, evening, or night to try to make sleep happen that night. While there is a lot you can do to set the stage for good sleep to happen in the long term, your efforts to make sleep happen on an immediate basis don't work and prolong your suffering.

☑ **Sleep efforts don't work.**

- In making sleep efforts, you are trying to control a passive process that you don't have conscious control over.

- Sleep efforts activate your nervous system at night by reinforcing the notion that a threat is present that must be battled through effort. To get past insomnia, you must learn how to get out of the way and let sleep happen on its own.

- Sleep efforts lead to additional frustration, confusion, and anxiety when they don't work, making it even harder to sleep.

- Sleep efforts can create psychological dependence, making you think you need to do all kinds of things during the day and night to sleep when you actually do not.

- Sleep efforts include actively doing things to try to make sleep happen as well as avoiding certain activities or stimuli out of fear that they will disrupt your sleep.

☑ **While it's generally a good idea to avoid screens before bed, don't worry about this too much.** Many normal sleepers use screens before bed all the time, and it doesn't cause them insomnia.

☑ **Only the *sleep-starting force and sleep-stopping force* control your sleep,** so work to let go of your sleep efforts. Sleep efforts make sleep way more complicated than it needs to be—and they actually amplify your sleep-stopping force.

CHAPTER

6

The Problems with CBT-i

Many insomnia sufferers have tried—or think they should try—Cognitive Behavioral Therapy for insomnia (CBT-i).

NOTE:
If you have no interest in CBT-i, feel free to skip ahead to Part 2—and start learning the End Insomnia System!

In the last chapter, you learned about why sleep efforts don't work—and how many advertised insomnia fixes fall under this umbrella. Building on this understanding, this chapter will examine why the primary therapeutic approach for insomnia, CBT-i (Cognitive Behavioral Therapy for insomnia), is not a good fit for many people.

You'll also see how the End Insomnia System offers something radically different from CBT-i. My hope is that you'll emerge from this chapter with more confidence that you truly can overcome insomnia using the approach you now have in your hands, even if you have tried everything else without success.

CBT-i is called the "gold standard" insomnia treatment by many reputable institutions. While research supports that CBT-i works for some people, many fall through the cracks or find that CBT-i does not bring a complete and permanent end to their insomnia.

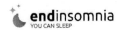

Let's examine the mechanisms that underlie CBT-i and how these compare to the End Insomnia System.

Breaking Down CBT-i: Sleep Education

First, CBT-i uses education to correct common misconceptions about sleep and provide an accurate understanding of how sleep works. Sleep education is a good thing. When you can't sleep and don't understand what's going on, it's easy to jump to false conclusions that can make the situation feel more alarming. Sleep education helps address this issue.

As part of the education process, many CBT-i practitioners recommend following "sleep hygiene" guidelines that are aimed at helping you achieve better sleep. Sleep hygiene lists often include things like:

+ Making your sleep environment cool, dark, quiet, and comfortable.
+ Avoiding blue light in the evening.
+ Avoiding caffeine, alcohol, and big meals too close to bedtime.
+ Following a specific pre-bedtime routine to prepare to sleep.
+ Getting exercise during the day so you are more tired at bedtime.
+ Getting morning light to help set your circadian rhythm.

While following sleep hygiene guidelines can help set the stage for better sleep, anxious people with insomnia get their hands on a sleep hygiene list and *militantly apply everything in a rigid way.* Then they still can't sleep and feel confused and *more* anxious.

Following a sleep hygiene checklist does not magically make you sleep and will not address your anxiety. If someone with insomnia gets too attached to sleep hygiene "working" for them, it will only add to their stress. This caveat is missing from some CBT-i protocols.

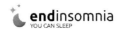

■ What's Different About the End Insomnia System's Approach to Sleep Education

As with CBT-i, proper knowledge about how sleep works is a core part of the End Insomnia System. However, the End Insomnia System places special emphasis on teaching how anxiety drives insomnia—and we offer unique and innovative tools to address that anxiety that are not a part of CBT-i. You'll learn all of these in Part 2 of the book.

Regarding sleep hygiene, we take a non-rigid approach. Following sleep hygiene guidelines is generally a good idea because it can help set the stage for sleep. For example, having good enough bedroom conditions is advisable, and you will probably have trouble sleeping if you're drinking coffee in the evening. However, we also make it clear that the real work is reducing sleep anxiety— not following a checklist of rules.

We also emphasize that following sleep hygiene guidelines can become an unhelpful sleep effort if you're not careful. For example, it's not helpful for someone with insomnia to believe they have no chance of sleeping unless they run five miles every day, or that their sleep will be ruined if they don't immediately go outside when they first wake up to get some natural light.

Using the End Insomnia System, you will eventually get to the point where you can follow some common sense sleep hygiene guidelines, but you won't overthink them. You can attain the casual relationship to sleep that a normal sleeper has, where you are not analyzing everything you do for the possible impacts it could have on your sleep that night.

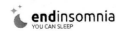

Breaking Down CBT-i: Cognitive Restructuring (to Manage Anxious Thoughts)

CBT-i uses cognitive restructuring (also known as thought challenging) as a core means of attempting to reduce sleep anxiety. Thought challenging is based on the idea that our worrisome thoughts are sometimes based on inaccurate assumptions.

Noticing anxious thoughts based on inaccurate assumptions and challenging those thoughts can at times bring relief. However, there are risks and limitations to this practice.

First, thought challenging can be used as an unhelpful sleep effort. Desperately trying to fight your thoughts at night to calm down and sleep is often a recipe for increased anxiety. If thought challenging can be done without it becoming a sleep effort, it can be helpful. You'll learn how in Chapter 10.

Second, if you believe you must talk yourself out of all your anxiety by thought challenging, you may be disappointed—or perhaps relieved—to learn that this is impossible. Although sometimes you may engage in extreme or catastrophic thinking about your insomnia, your anxiety about insomnia will often be based on the truth: you are in a difficult situation that you have limited control over.

If you are anxious that if you don't get to sleep soon, you will likely have to deal with consequences like fatigue and a lower mood the next day, your thinking is based in reality.

While it makes sense to challenge an extreme thought such as "I won't be able to survive tomorrow if I don't get to sleep soon," the truth is, the next day could indeed be hard, and it makes sense that you might be anxious about it. There are realities of the insomnia experience that are natural to feel anxious about, and you will not always be able to talk yourself out of that anxiety.

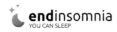

A risk of thought challenging is that if it doesn't work, you might feel like a failure or like it is your fault that you can't fully talk yourself out of your anxiety. Insomnia inevitably involves anxiety. It's inescapable, and we don't always need to fight it with thought challenging.

■ What's Different About the End Insomnia System's Approach to Managing Anxious Thoughts

Thought challenging has its place in the End Insomnia System, as you'll learn in Chapter 10. Sometimes it's the best way to ease anxiety. However, over-emphasizing thought challenging in the process of overcoming insomnia is a big mistake.

Because sometimes your anxiety will be grounded in the difficult reality of your situation or because you simply cannot seem to talk yourself out of your anxiety, it's crucial to have the ability to accept worrisome thoughts—and learn to hold them more lightly.

You'll learn about these new ways to relate to your thoughts throughout Part 2—beginning in Chapter 9. As you'll see, there are times when you must accept the reality of your present situation and learn how to be less reactive in the face of uncertainty and poor sleep. In doing so, you will stop inadvertently feeding your anxiety—and learn unexpected ways that your anxiety can be reduced.

This core approach to managing anxious insomnia thoughts is missing from traditional CBT-i.

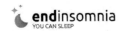

Breaking Down CBT-i: Relaxation Training

Some CBT-i practitioners also incorporate various relaxation training techniques into the treatment. For example, this could be breathing exercises, progressive muscle relaxation, or meditation. Learning how to regulate your nervous system using these sorts of techniques is helpful.

The risk is that if you are not carefully instructed in the intention behind using such techniques, you are liable to use them as short-term sleep efforts that will let you down and leave you frustrated.

■ What's Different About the End Insomnia System's Approach

The End Insomnia System draws upon some nervous system regulation tools like meditation; however, our instructions about why you are doing the practice are crystal clear. It is not to make yourself sleep (because sleep efforts don't work.) Rather the intention behind using these tools is long-term reconditioning of your nervous system.

Tools like these are one of many ways the End Insomnia System works to gradually lower your sleep-stopping force. The intention you bring to nervous system regulation practices makes all the difference in whether they help you or just leave you confused and disappointed.

Additionally, in our approach, tools like meditation are not just aimed at learning how to "relax." Rather, they are used to build a new set of skills to address your insomnia on a deeper level. Meditation trains your mind to be less reactive and more flexible toward the experiences of life that you don't have full control over (which is extremely relevant for the journey through insomnia). You'll learn much more about this later in the book.

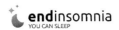

Breaking Down CBT-i: Behavioral Interventions

The primary mechanism of change in CBT-i is two intense behavioral rules known as *sleep restriction and stimulus control*. Both are meant to retrain your body to sleep. Let's break them down.

■ Sleep Restriction

With sleep restriction, you limit your time in bed each night to the amount you are currently sleeping on average. This might mean giving yourself only a five- or six-hour opportunity to sleep each night—which can feel very extreme if you need closer to seven or eight hours of sleep to feel restored.

This restricted sleep schedule is kept up for multiple weeks. For some, restricting their time in bed in this way often leads to additional anxiety that makes it even harder to sleep—because there is extra pressure to *SLEEP NOW!* when you have such limited time in bed.

The intent, though, is to create sleep deprivation to the point that your body's biological drive to sleep is powerful enough to force sleep to happen. When your body is so exhausted that sleep happens even in the presence of anxiety, the hope is that you begin to regain confidence in the process of falling asleep and staying asleep.

This sleep restriction regimen is paired with:

■ Stimulus Control

Stimulus control involves attempting to reassociate being in bed to sleeping quickly, as opposed to lying there awake. The idea is that the more you experience getting into bed and falling asleep quickly, the more your mind will be reconditioned to expect this to happen, and it will happen more and more frequently.

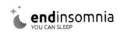

First, to implement stimulus control, you avoid being in your bed and, ideally, even your bedroom, for anything but sleep or sex.

Second, you are instructed to get out of bed if you don't fall asleep within 20 or 30 minutes.

When you get out of bed, you're instructed to go do something relaxing until you're feeling sleepy again and then return to bed and see if sleep happens. If you don't fall asleep within 20 or 30 minutes, you leave your bed again. Again, the hope is that if you are not spending a long time awake in bed, you retrain your brain to expect to sleep when you go to bed rather than to lie awake for hours.

■ Where Sleep Restriction and Stimulus Control Go Wrong

In principle, the ideas behind sleep restriction and stimulus control make sense. However, some people who try to implement these techniques find that they end up increasing their sleep anxiety and do not provide a long-term solution to insomnia. Let's explore why.

As for sleep restriction, many people find that spending such a short amount of time in bed causes a significant amount of additional anxiety that makes them feel more broken and desperate. I've talked to many people who share my view that the CBT-i approach to sleep restriction does not feel like a reasonable or sustainable solution. This is especially true if, after one grueling multi-week round of sleep restriction, you are instructed to start sleep restriction all over again when your poor sleep and sleep anxiety return (which they often do).

Regarding stimulus control, for many, the procedure of getting in and out of bed when they can't sleep creates more anxiety. People following stimulus control guidelines often lie in bed feeling nervous about having to get up again if they don't sleep soon. In an effort to comply with the rule, they may lie in bed, anxious and preoccupied, estimating how much time has passed and whether they need to get out of bed again.

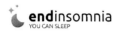

Although stimulus control aims to recondition the brain to associate bed with sleep, it can also inadvertently create new associations in your brain between sleep and overthinking what you must do for sleep to happen. Unless you have a calm and flexible attitude about following stimulus control guidelines (which typically does not describe your average person with insomnia), then stimulus control can lead you to believe that you need to follow rigid and unnatural rules if you want to be able to sleep. For many, this has the net negative effect of pulling you further away from a normal, low-stakes, flexible relationship to sleep and your bed.

I've heard from a range of people about how CBT-i techniques can go awry. If you've tried it, here's a pretty typical example of how it may have gone:

When you hired a therapist to help you use CBT-I, you restricted your time in bed to the point where even if you slept through the entire allotted time (which is pretty unlikely to happen), you knew you'd still feel awful the next day. Knowing that there wasn't any possible way to get enough sleep to feel rested, you felt additional anxiety that made it harder to sleep.

Using your sleep-restricted schedule, you may have found yourself unable to sleep and getting out of bed within 30 minutes of attempting to sleep. You may have sat up in the middle of the night, feeling absolute despair that *these were the tools there were supposed to help you sleep.*

After some time passed, you returned to bed. There, you waited again to see if you would need to get out of bed again—while hoping your sleep drive would overpower the increasing anxiety you felt as you implemented these rigid behavioral guidelines.

You may remember feeling paranoid during the day if you went anywhere close to your bed because you worried about messing up the CBT-I rule of avoiding the bed and bedroom for anything but sleep and sex. It can feel like entering your bedroom during the day is jeopardizing your ability to reclaim the normal sleep you longed for.

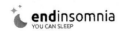

However, when you stuck with these behavioral rules over the course of weeks (you were willing to do virtually anything to get better sleep again), your sleep may have actually begun to improve. You found yourself falling asleep more quickly and staying asleep for much of the night. Even though you still weren't getting enough sleep, this was quite a relief. You were hopeful that this was a sign that your insomnia was almost behind you.

Unfortunately, like many people find, within a few weeks of stopping CBT-I, your sleep deteriorated to where it was before. However, you now felt much more broken and hopeless because the supposed "best treatment" had failed you.

So you began to dread that you would have to do this painful multi-week regimen of CBT-i again and again for the rest of your life. It seemed incomprehensible, but it was your only option at the time.

■ What's Different About the End Insomnia System's Approach to Behavioral Guidelines

Now, let's talk about the End Insomnia System's response to the issues that some people encounter with CBT-i. This approach believes in the importance of having a strong sleep-starting force. A critical part of the End Insomnia system is following a set of realistic and sustainable guidelines that you will be able to keep over the long term to optimize your sleep-starting force.

Following our gentle guidelines does not have the same risk of increased anxiety that comes with CBT-i's hardcore sleep restriction. You'll learn these guidelines in Chapter 8.

Unlike CBT-i's sleep restriction, this approach does not place as much emphasis on creating an extremely high sleep-starting force as the central mechanism of change.

Instead, we believe that once you have a strong-enough sleep-starting force (sleep drive and circadian rhythm), the real work is to lower the sleep-stopping force (anxiety and hyperarousal).

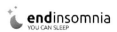

Here's the *crucial* element of overcoming insomnia that CBT-i sometimes neglects: In order to lower your sleep anxiety, it's not enough to show yourself that you can sleep *under certain conditions*—**you need to become less afraid of the experience and consequences of your insomnia.**

This idea is at the core of the End Insomnia System.

Our aim is to help you feel more okay and less threatened—no matter how you sleep. The system provides a powerful set of tools, perspectives, and knowledge to reach this goal. Using this book, you can truly become less attached to how you sleep, meaning there's less performance anxiety and fear to keep you awake in the first place.

Following CBT-i's rigid stimulus control and sleep restriction guidelines may help you sleep, but in some cases, it just covers over your underlying sleep anxiety by forcing your body into exhaustion-induced sleep.

In the End Insomnia System, we examine your sleep anxiety from all angles— and disassemble it permanently.

Concluding Thoughts on CBT-i

While CBT-i definitely works for some people, others find that it makes their situation worse. For people who are highly anxious about not sleeping and the consequences, it's easy to see how CBT-i has the potential to amp up their anxiety. Even if it works temporarily by retraining your body to sleep, CBT-i often does not thoroughly address the root cause: anxiety about not sleeping and the consequences. If this anxiety is just temporarily covered over rather than fundamentally addressed, there is a high chance insomnia will eventually resurface.

Drawing on newer modalities of psychological change, the End Insomnia System offers a different approach to overcoming insomnia, strongly focused on targeting and resolving sleep anxiety.

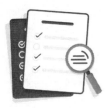

KEY CHAPTER TAKEAWAYS

☑   CBT-i works for some people, but many find it does not fix their insomnia, and some find it actually worsens their problem.

☑   The core mechanisms of change in CBT-i are behavioral guidelines known as sleep restriction and stimulus control. These focus on retraining you to sleep through intense behavioral changes made to induce sleep, but may not be effective at addressing the underlying anxiety that stops you from sleeping in the first place.

☑   The End Insomnia System balances sustainable behavioral changes to create a reasonably strong sleep-starting force (sleep drive and circadian rhythm) while putting the main focus on reducing the sleep-stopping force (anxiety and hyperarousal) that gets in the way of effortless sleep happening.

Part 2

The End Insomnia System

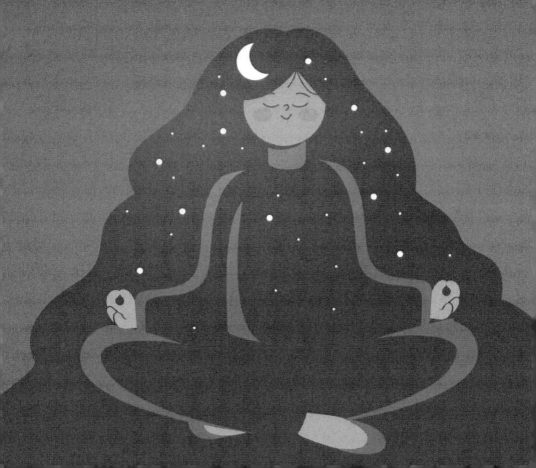

CHAPTER

7

The Way to End Insomnia

It's time to talk about what the End Insomnia System is—and how it can help you permanently end your insomnia.

The End Insomnia System takes a two-pronged approach:

+ *Raising your **sleep-starting force.***
+ *Lowering your **sleep-stopping force.***

These are the *only* two things you have to do.

The rest of Part 2 will show you how.

First, we'll address the sleep-starting force. Remember, this consists of two natural components—your sleep drive and your circadian rhythm.

No matter how long you've struggled with insomnia or how bad you feel it is, your sleep-starting force is still there—waiting for you to strengthen it.

You'll get a simple way to do just that next, in Chapter 8: *A Simple Way to Kickstart Your Journey to Better Sleep.*

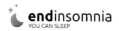
The chapters that follow shift the focus to lowering your **sleep-stopping force**—the anxiety and hyperarousal that keep you locked in a vicious cycle of insomnia:

+ *Mindful Acceptance (Chapter 9)*

+ *Managing Anxious Thoughts (Chapter 10)*

+ *What to Do at Night When You Can't Get to Sleep (Chapter 11)*

+ *Finding Daytime Resilience When Fatigued (Chapter 12)*

+ *Self-Compassion (Chapter 13)*

+ *Meditation (Chapter 14)*

+ *Mindsets to Accelerate Your Progress (Chapter 15)*

+ *Finding Appropriate Support (Chapter 16)*

When you apply what you learn in Part 2, you will boost your sleep-starting force and lower your sleep-stopping force—and over time, resolve your insomnia so you can get consistent natural sleep without any effort.

Setting Expectations

You don't become entrenched in the vicious cycle of insomnia in a single night. The anxiety; the unhelpful perceptions, reactions, and behaviors; and the conditioned hyperarousal get built up and reinforced over time.

Since insomnia doesn't develop overnight, you also can't expect an overnight solution (not a lasting one, anyway).

The End Insomnia System is not a quick fix. The process of calming the underlying anxiety and changing the factors that drive insomnia takes time. The system in this book is a **long-term solution** that requires you to learn how to face and manage your discomfort—and accept the reality that in the process of getting to long-term great sleep, you will have to go through numerous ups and downs in your sleep and emotional experience.

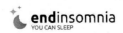
This approach requires persistence, patience, learning new things, and facing uncomfortable experiences. It involves learning what you can control—and what you cannot.

The End Insomnia System is not as easy as taking a pill. But it's a lot more effective—and empowering.

And if you're already trapped in the suffering of insomnia, isn't it worth committing to something that might take some work—but can finally free you?

■ How long does it take?

It is very natural to wonder how long this process will take to deliver results. I have heard people say that even if they knew for sure that their insomnia would be gone in, say, six months, they would feel enormous relief in the meantime.

Unfortunately, there is no guaranteed timeline for getting results from this system. The speed of the process varies from person to person.

While you may experience relief and some swift changes as you start to apply the knowledge and tools in this book, it often takes a couple of months of consistent practice to see lasting change.

For people who have had insomnia for many years or who have had an especially traumatic time with it, sometimes it can take longer, for example, six months, or even more.

But if you stick with it, you can get there. And sometimes, the people who have had the "worst" insomnia move past it surprisingly quickly—it depends on many factors and cannot be easily predicted.

The best practice is to let go of the timeline for this process. The more closely you monitor your progress, the more anxiety you will create—which will just get in the way.

Make your intention just to take it one day at a time. Try to appreciate the journey. While it's not easy, it is interesting. It's all about YOU, after all.

Things to Know Before You Start

As we covered in Part 1, *the root cause of ongoing insomnia is deeply ingrained anxiety about not sleeping.* To begin to soften that anxiety, let's correct some common misconceptions:

■ How Much Sleep Do I Need?

The first common source of anxiety for many with insomnia is the popular notion that you need eight hours of sleep. You may have seen or heard sources claiming that you are harming your health if you don't get eight hours of sleep.

The truth is that we all have unique sleep needs. There are many people whose bodies simply don't need eight hours of sleep to feel refreshed. For these people, it is futile to arbitrarily attempt to reach eight hours of sleep.

I've known people with naturally lower sleep needs who initially developed insomnia because they tried to make themselves get eight hours. They spent long periods awake at night, which planted seeds of doubt about sleep in their minds. They began to overthink sleep and develop sleep anxiety—which started the vicious cycle. Before long, they had ongoing insomnia.

If you are not someone who needs eight hours of sleep, there is nothing wrong with you.

The National Sleep Foundation determined that 7–9 hours is the average sleep needed for the average adult—but as few as 6 hours is enough for some people. For those over 65, the foundation determined that 7–8 hours is the average sleep need, but that as few as 5 hours of sleep is appropriate for some.

When you come out on the other side of insomnia, you will likely get about as much sleep as you used to get. The takeaway is to not hold yourself to an arbitrary standard of sleep need. Doing so can make your sleep anxiety worse.

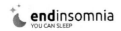

One easy way to tell roughly how much sleep your body needs is to see how many hours of sleep lets you (1) feel reasonably refreshed when you wake up, and (2) have good energy for most of the day.

After having insomnia for a while, it can be easy to have perfectionistic ideals of what good sleep is—perhaps that "good sleep" equals "feeling good all day." Remember that normal sleepers also have ups and downs in their energy throughout the day. Many don't feel amazing when they first wake up. And even with normal sleep, most people experience an afternoon "crash" due to circadian rhythms.

As long as you have decent energy for much of the day, you're getting enough sleep.

■ Insomnia Won't Kill You—or Ruin Your Health

A major cause of sleep-related anxiety is fear about the health implications of insomnia. There is a lot of misinformation on this issue—and many sensationalized headlines that don't represent the facts.

First off, let's talk about the lack of evidence that insomnia increases your risk of death. A 2018 meta-analysis of 17 studies examined chronic insomnia and mortality, spanning almost 37 million individuals who were checked on for an average of 11.6 years.

The meta-analysis found no difference in the odds of mortality for individuals with insomnia symptoms compared to those without.

There are many reasons to be skeptical of correlation studies making claims about the health effects of insomnia. First, correlation does not prove causation. Insomnia has never been shown to cause any health problems.

There are some correlations between insomnia and conditions like cardiovascular disease and Alzheimer's—but correlation is not causation. Just because two things may happen together does not mean that one caused the other.

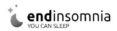

Rather than insomnia causing certain diseases, it is reasonable to imagine that people with Alzheimer's or cardiovascular disease may have more trouble sleeping because of those conditions themselves, not because poor sleep brought on those diseases.

Furthermore, sleep research often relies on inaccurate self-report data, small sample sizes, or low thresholds of statistical significance that make reproducing and validating the findings difficult. For these reasons, it is worth taking sleep research with a grain of salt.

There is no final answer on the exact links between sleep and health; however, there is plenty of reason to believe that it's not as bad as headlines make it out to be. And worrying about the health impacts of poor sleep makes it even harder to break free from insomnia and have a calm nervous system at night.

If you are ready to leave your insomnia behind, then take the evidence that insomnia will not kill you and has not been proven to cause any health problems, let go of obsessing about sleep and health—and join me in Chapter 8.

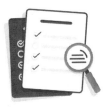

KEY CHAPTER TAKEAWAYS

☑ The End Insomnia System is not a quick fix. It's a process to help you overcome insomnia in the long term, so you can have good sleep for life.

☑ It requires patience, consistency, and a willingness to face discomfort. And it works.

☑ While it's natural to want to know how long the process will take, there is no guaranteed timeline. It's best to focus on the changes you are making rather than monitoring your progress.

☑ That said, most people see some results in the initial weeks—and much more after a few months.

☑ Misinformation about sleep and health is a source of added stress when working through insomnia.

☑ Not everyone requires eight hours of sleep. If you feel reasonably refreshed when you wake up and have good energy for most of the day, you're getting enough sleep.

☑ Once you address the factors that drive insomnia, you will likely get about as much sleep as you used to. For those who have had insomnia for a very long time and don't have a sense of what their body needs anymore, this method will lead you to get the right amount of sleep for your current needs.

☑ Even long-term insomnia has not been shown to increase the risk of death. Research has not shown that insomnia causes disease.

A Simple Way to Kickstart Your Journey to Better Sleep

Optimizing the Sleep-Starting Force by Using a "Sleep Window"

Let's start with something simple (not necessarily easy, just simple). While the majority of this book focuses on dialing down the sleep-stopping force, a quick and foundational step to end insomnia is to dial up the sleep-starting force.

You'll remember that what I call the **sleep-starting force** has two parts: Your sleep drive and your circadian rhythm. This chapter will cover creating and using a "sleep window"—a way to structure your sleep time—in a way that will optimize your sleep-starting force.

While you may have encountered the idea of a sleep window before, in contrast to some other insomnia protocols:

1. The sleep window structure we use is meant to be sustainable and realistic for the long term (unlike sleep windows used in, say, CBT-i, which are often very short and can cause extra anxiety).

2. In the End Insomnia System, we're very careful to help you understand that using a sleep window is not a sleep effort, but is rather a means of *boosting your sleep-starting force* to set the stage for long-term good sleep.

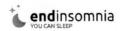

Following these guidelines consistently throughout your journey of overcoming insomnia ensures that your body's natural biological tendency to fall and stay asleep gives you all the help it can.

Your Sleep Window

The time you set aside as your opportunity to sleep at night is called your "sleep window." To establish your sleep window, you need to:

1. Spend the right amount of time in bed.

2. Get out of bed at about the same time every day.

3. Avoid long naps.

These are the three main guidelines. (Later in the chapter, I'll also give you some important DOs and DON'Ts.)

Before we explain these guidelines in detail, here's a brief overview of why each is important and what it does for you:

1. ***Spend the right amount of time in bed***—because the length of your sleep window affects your **sleep drive.**

2. ***Get out of bed at about the same time every day***—because the timing of your sleep window affects your **circadian rhythm.**

3. ***Avoid long naps***—because preserving your sleep window (and sleeping exclusively then) affects **both** your sleep drive and your circadian rhythm.

Let's break these down.

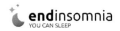

Sleep Window Length

Spending the right amount of time in bed is critical to ensure your **sleep drive** is primed to help you get to sleep.

Why this helps: It's obvious why too little time in bed would be a problem. But many people with insomnia spend too much time in bed—either by going to bed too early or by staying in bed well past when they would typically rise. Understandably, they want to allow themselves the chance to sleep more. But, ironically, spending too long in bed undermines your sleep by reinforcing the insomnia loop. Here's why:

For your sleep drive to be strong enough to support your ability to fall asleep and stay asleep, you need to be awake and active for enough hours during the day.

If you are in bed for more time than you need:

- ✦ You don't give your sleep drive adequate time to build during the day.
- ✦ You inevitably end up lying awake for long periods—which will confirm your fears about not being able to sleep.

You're probably familiar with the term "sleep debt" to refer to functioning on less than enough sleep. Well, your sleep drive can also be in "debt."

If you're spending an extra two hours in bed each night, you're creating two hours of sleep-drive debt—which means that your sleep drive is weaker (by two hours' worth) the next night.

If you instead spend those two hours awake and active, you raise your sleep drive (two hours' worth). Two hours—even one hour—of extra built-up sleep drive can make a huge difference in your ability to fall and stay asleep.

Why this is necessary: Even if you lower your sleep-stopping force by utilizing the tools in every other chapter of this book *if you are not optimizing your*

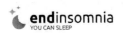
biological sleep drive by spending the right amount of time in bed, your progress toward improved sleep will likely flounder. You will wonder why your efforts to reduce your anxiety are not leading to the results you want.

So only spend as much time in bed as the amount of sleep you would need to feel reasonably refreshed and have decent energy throughout your day.

How to determine the length of your sleep window: If you remember how much you used to sleep before you had insomnia, or you know how much sleep you generally need to feel refreshed, aim for that number of hours as your sleep window.

You want a sleep window that will be sustainable long term. It's crucial not to exaggerate how long you should spend in bed.

Here's an example. Let's say you need 8 hours of sleep to feel rested. That means that out of 24 hours in a day, you'll need to be awake for 16 hours to have an adequately high sleep drive to enable you to sleep for most of your sleep window the next night. (If you need 7 hours of sleep to feel rested, you need to be active for 17 hours...and so forth.)

While spending a specified time in bed may spark some initial anxiety, this is the **only way to prime the sleep drive** to help you overcome ongoing insomnia. You need your sleep biology to be on your side through this process.

If a temporary rise in anxiety leads to worse sleep at first, know that this problem is self-correcting: The sleep deficit will create a stronger sleep drive in the coming nights. It won't be long before your higher sleep drive forces sleep to happen—even if you have a lot of anxiety.

It may take a bit of experimentation over several weeks to get your sleep window right. Monitor if the sleep window you are using leads you to feel consistently sleepy around bedtime.

If you are consistently sleepy around bedtime, this is a good sign that your sleep window is helping to give you a strong sleep drive. If you are consistently not very sleepy around bedtime, it may be a sign that your sleep window is too long.

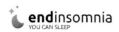

How to give your sleep drive an even bigger "bio boost": If you want to give yourself extra sleep-starting help from your own biology, then give yourself a little less time in bed than you think you need.

If you want to try this, start with about 30 minutes less than you think you need. Having *a slightly shorter sleep window can help kick your sleep drive into a higher gear* and increase your chances of sleep. And an extra-high sleep drive early in your process of working through insomnia can help build your confidence— and inspire you to keep going.

However, ultimately, you want a sleep window that you are comfortable sticking to long term. The sleep window guidelines of the End Insomnia System are intended to be sustainable and realistic, not extreme like the sleep restriction intervention prescribed by CBT-i.

Sleep Window Timing (Get Out of Bed at About the Same Time Every Day)

The second sleep-window guideline is to get out of bed (i.e., end your sleep window) at about the **same time every day.**

Why does this help? This is important because it helps set your **circadian rhythm** (the other part of the sleep-starting force). Doing this will help your body experience sleepiness and wakefulness in a predictable pattern that will support easeful sleep.

Getting up at the same time each day also helps to enforce your sleep window so you do not sabotage your sleep drive by lying around in bed in the morning.

Choose to get up at a time that works best for your life. I highly recommend using an alarm to help you stick to your wake time. (And don't hit "snooze"!)

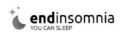

Try not to deviate from your wake time by more than 20 or 30 minutes, even on weekends or vacations. Setting your circadian rhythm is done over the course of weeks, so sticking to your wake-up time consistently is an investment in your future good sleep.

(If there is a very occasional morning in which you sleep in for an hour because you were out late, that is okay, but too many deviations from your wake time can set back your progress.)

If you're someone who wakes prematurely before your sleep window ends, I encourage you to remain in bed and give yourself the opportunity to possibly fall back asleep until the end of your sleep window. If you feel miserable lying in bed and feel that you must get up, that's okay too.

You won't need to maintain a consistent sleep window forever—but when working through insomnia and rebuilding confidence in your sleep, you want all the forces of sleep biology on your side. A sleep window is an important step toward improved sleep.

How to schedule your sleep window: Set your exact sleep window by counting back the number of hours in your sleep window length from your desired wake-up time. For example, let's say you need a seven-hour sleep window, and you have to get up at 6 a.m. Then your sleep window would be from 11 p.m to 6 a.m.

Getting up at the same time each day is difficult when you have not slept well, but it is doable—especially when you apply the psychological tools and perspectives you will learn later in this book.

So commit to getting up at the same time each day and persist through any anxiety it brings. Regulating your circadian rhythm is an important way to dial up your sleep-starting force.

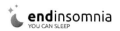

A NOTE ON SHIFT WORK

If you are a shift worker and your schedule fluctuates, you may not be able to apply these guidelines exactly as directed. Do your best to apply the guidelines around the schedule constraints you have.

If you can't fully apply these guidelines due to your schedule, you can still do your best to ensure your sleep drive is high when you go to sleep. You can also still do plenty to reduce the sleep-stopping force of anxiety and hyperarousal (the focus of the rest of the book after this chapter).

Preserve Your Sleep Window (Avoid Long Naps)

Preserve and enhance your sleep window by avoiding long naps. The process of overcoming insomnia is easier if you sleep only in your sleep window.

Why does this help? Naps undermine the good work you are doing by:

+ Reducing your **sleep drive** for the night ahead.
+ Throwing off your **circadian rhythm.**

So a long nap can sabotage *both* parts of your **sleep-starting force**!

Generally speaking, it's best to avoid napping at all. However, if you really feel the need, or if you actually find yourself falling asleep during your day, then a short nap is okay.

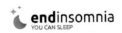
If you do nap, limit it to **30 minutes** and have it **before 3 p.m.** to minimize interference with your sleep for that night. Be sure to set an alarm so you don't oversleep.

If you try to nap and can't fall asleep, just close your eyes and rest. Simply resting for 20 or 30 minutes is restorative. This can set a better tone for the rest of your day.

Easing Into Your Sleep Window: DOs and DON'Ts

■ DOS: Have a Low-Pressure Wind-Down

A low-pressure wind-down 45–60 minutes before the start of your sleep window helps you shift from the activity and busyness of the day to a more settled and sleep-compatible nervous system state.

Unlike pre-bedtime sleep efforts, this wind-down is **not intended to make sleep happen.** Rather than getting attached to your wind-down creating a certain outcome tonight, just let it be something you do that can support easeful sleep in the long term—and can be an enjoyable end to your day. Choose an activity that you enjoy for its own sake. You could read, listen to music or a podcast, or watch something you enjoy. You could meditate (as long as you're not meditating as a sleep effort). You could relax with your family or do some art.

While you may choose to avoid blue light in the evening to give extra support to your circadian rhythm, it's not a big deal to watch a show or movie if you find that's a good way for you to relax at night. This is something many normal sleepers do. Remember, anxiety is the real problem here, not blue light.

As you anticipate the night ahead, you might be quite keyed up and anxious before bed. For this reason, it's normal if your wind-down is not totally calm and peaceful. However, having a wind-down gives you a way to **focus on something you enjoy,** so you are less likely to focus on anxious rumination as bedtime approaches.

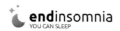

If anxious thoughts arise during your wind-down, that's no problem. Just do your best to keep your attention on the activity in front of you rather than on the anxious thoughts. You will learn more strategies for managing anxious thoughts in Chapter 10.

■ DON'T: Don't Watch the Clock

If you feel preoccupied and anxious after you begin your wind-down, then a helpful strategy is to **stop watching the clock when you start your wind-down** and just go to bed whenever you feel sleepy. If this is a bit before or a bit after the official start of your sleep window, that's okay.

This strategy helps you remove any clock-induced pressure from your wind-down routine so you can focus more on being present with your wind-down activity. When you aren't obsessively watching the clock, it will be easier and more natural to notice the cues from your body about when it's time to sleep.

■ DON'T: Don't Try to Force Sleep

Here's another key way to avoid turning your sleep window into a sleep effort: If you're not sleepy at the start of your sleep window, **don't try to force it.** Sleepy is different from tired-but-wired. Sleepiness includes physiological signs such as yawning, drooping eyelids or nodding off.

Instead of trying to force sleep, accept that you are not yet sleepy—and accept that the best thing to do is to stay awake until you truly are.

There are two options for following this guideline. First, you can choose to stay out of bed until you are truly sleepy. Do something that you find pleasant and relaxing, such as reading a book, listening to a podcast, or watching something until you feel more sleepy.

When you feel truly sleepy, then go to bed. Staying up until you are sleepy doesn't guarantee you will fall asleep quickly, but it increases the chances that you will, which is helpful for regaining confidence that you can sleep.

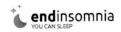

Some find that staying up out of bed past the start of their sleep window causes them extra anxiety. So the second option is to go to bed at the start of your sleep window—but allow yourself to stay awake in bed until sleepy.

Again, you can read, listen to something, watch something, or just rest and relax as best you can until you are truly sleepy. The point here is just to be flexible if you are not sleepy and to accept having more time awake if sleep doesn't seem to be happening. Having a plan of what you'll do if you are not sleepy helps to avoid frustration and unhelpful reactivity that can make you even more awake.

Both of these options are ways to make peace with the fact that you cannot force sleep to happen. While it can be anxiety-producing to reach the start of your sleep window and not feel sleepy, this is not something you have full control over. The best you can do is to occupy yourself until your body is in a more sleep-compatible state—and not make the situation worse by using sleep efforts.

Concluding Thoughts on Your Sleep Window

While implementing a sleep window may lead to a temporary increase in anxiety, remember that this is just a phase. As you adjust to these guidelines, you won't feel so anxious about them, and you will begin to see how they bring you closer to being a normal sleeper again—and how they help you fall asleep and stay asleep more easily.

Some people resist following these guidelines—but without them, your journey through insomnia will be much slower, more complicated, and more confusing.

These guidelines are meant to be sustainable and realistic. Yes, it will be hard to stick with these guidelines at times—but insomnia is hard regardless. If you do not follow these guidelines, you will likely experience greater hardship in the long term than if you stick to them and overcome the short-term discomfort of adjusting to them.

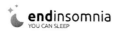

If limiting your time in bed in these ways feels too daunting right now, then implement a sleep window after you learn some of the other tools in the later chapters. The rest of the End Insomnia System will help soothe your anxiety and make you feel more empowered and resilient regardless of how you sleep.

If you want guidance, support, and accountability in implementing and sticking to these foundational behavioral guidelines to overcome your insomnia, the coaches and community at the **End Insomnia Program** can help. Speed up your journey through insomnia by getting things right from the start.

JOIN US AT:

https://endinsomnia.com/program

KEY CHAPTER TAKEAWAYS

☑ **To increase your sleep-starting force,** stick to the following guidelines:

☑ **DO: Create a Sleep Window**

- **Spend the right amount of time in bed.** Make it equal to the number of hours you would need to sleep to feel pretty rested. More time in bed undercuts your **sleep drive** (part of the **sleep-starting force**) and gets in the way of reclaiming long-term good sleep.

- **Get up at the same time every day.** This sets your **circadian rhythm** (part of the **sleep-starting force**) to help you feel sleepy and awake at appropriate times.

- **Avoid long naps.** Naps can mess with your sleep-starting force.It's best to skip naps entirely, but if you must take a short nap, limit it to 30 minutes before 3 p.m.

☑ **DOS:Have a low-pressure wind-down.** Do something relaxing you enjoy for its own sake for your wind-down. Don't make it a sleep effort. If you find you are anxiously watching the clock during your window, stop looking at your clock at the start of your wind-down and just go to bed when you are sleepy.

☑ **DON'T: Watch the clock.** When you start your wind-down, stop watching the clock and just go to bed when you're sleepy, whether that is a bit before or after the start of your sleep window. Tracking the time is counterproductive.

☑ **DON'T: Try to force sleep to happen.** If you reach the start of your sleep window and do not feel sleepy, do something relaxing (in or out of bed) to occupy your mind until you feel more sleepy. This can help you find more peace with what is and prevent you from lying in bed trying to make yourself sleep (which doesn't work and doesn't help).

CHAPTER 9

Mindful Acceptance

Lowering the Sleep-Stopping Force by Reducing Reactivity

The last chapter focused on simple ways to boost your sleep-starting force. As promised, we will now turn our attention to lowering the **sleep-stopping force.**

Again, what I refer to as the **sleep-stopping force** is the *anxiety* and *hyperarousal* that keep your body wired—and awake—even when the biological conditions for sleep are otherwise present.

Insomnia causes a huge amount of discomfort. It is frightening and can make you feel trapped and out of control. Yet there are steps you can take to make it more bearable. Here's a secret:

Sleeping well consistently comes from **caring less about sleeping well.**

I get that this might sound unattainable. But bear with me. It is possible to *learn how to manage and reduce the distress* that poor sleep causes.

You can train your mind and nervous system to be more calm and more flexible when you experience sleep troubles—or any other adversity in your life. You can train yourself to care less.

Why reducing reactivity helps. When you find greater indifference to how you sleep, your nervous system will be much calmer at night and will be in a more sleep-compatible state.

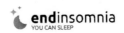

When you can find ways to care less about how you sleep, it is also easier to stick to the guidelines from Chapter 8 that increase your sleep-starting force and accelerate your progress through insomnia.

This chapter will teach you to use **mindful acceptance** to become more resilient (and feel less miserable) when you do sleep poorly. This is one of the foundational ways the End Insomnia System helps you lower your sleep-stopping force.

Mindful Acceptance: Mindfulness + Acceptance

Mindful acceptance, as the name implies, combines mindfulness and acceptance. First, let's talk about what we mean by mindfulness.

Mindfulness: Mindfulness is simply the ability to recognize what is happening in the present moment with an open attitude (again, simply—not necessarily easily... especially at first. Which is why we make mindfulness a practice).

When you are mindful, you are not caught up in daydreams or wandering thoughts—you are right here, right now.

Mindfulness allows you to recognize when you are caught in an unhelpful struggle against your thoughts, feelings, or sensations—and then shift into a stance of acceptance.

Jon Kabat-Zinn, who pioneered mindfulness-based stress reduction in the West, defines mindfulness as "the awareness that arises when we pay attention, on purpose, in the present moment, and non-judgmentally."

Mindfulness helps us do five things:

+ Have clear and non-judgmental awareness of what's happening right now.

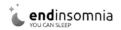

- ✦ Step back from over-identifying with thoughts and feelings.

- ✦ Respond intentionally to what is happening, rather than reacting in an unconscious or habitual way.

- ✦ Be present and fully engaged with whatever we're doing.

- ✦ Slow down so we can be *curious* about our experience and question why we are thinking, feeling, or reacting the way we are.

Mindfulness is important because we often go through the day on autopilot. Normally this isn't a huge problem: We all have habits and patterns that we use to help us navigate our lives.

However, running on autopilot becomes a *major problem* when we're stuck in the cycle of insomnia. Without bringing a greater level of awareness to what is happening—and then choosing to respond in new ways—it is difficult to break out of the vicious cycle of anxiety that drives insomnia.

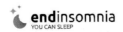
MINDFULNESS EXERCISE: AWARENESS OF THE BREATH

To get a quick taste of the experience of mindfulness, try this exercise.

Sit up straight, breathe normally, and begin to notice your breathing. Focus on the sensation of breathing: the rise and fall of your belly, or the feeling of air passing in and out of your nostrils. Choose whatever sensation is easiest for you to notice.

Now, just for the next three minutes, place your attention on the sensation of your breath. Use a timer so you can free your attention from the passing of time.

During this three-minute experiment, simply watch the inflow and outflow of the breath. Your breath is always happening in the present, so paying attention to the breath is a way to keep your attention anchored in the present.

As you are doing this exercise, it's normal for your mind to wander. Just try to notice when this has happened and then return your attention to the breath

Ready? Set a timer and go.

*

Hopefully, you were able to stay with the sensation of your breath for a good portion of the three minutes. That's a taste of what it feels like to have your attention in the present moment.

In the previous exercise, you used your breath as the focus of your awareness— but you can apply mindful awareness to whatever you experience. You can apply mindfulness to:

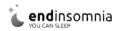

- ✦ Anything you perceive with your five senses.

- ✦ The thoughts you notice yourself thinking.

- ✦ Joyful, painful, or neutral emotions and how they feel in your body.

- ✦ Body sensations (pleasant or unpleasant).

- ✦ Any activity of life (preparing food, taking a walk, bathing, reading this book—or anything else).

While a simple mindfulness exercise like this may at first seem unrelated to overcoming your insomnia, the idea behind the exercise is simply to **practice building the mental muscle** of present-moment awareness.

Present-moment awareness—mindfulness—is the foundation for the second part of mindful acceptance: Acceptance.

Acceptance: Acceptance is related to mindfulness: You can only "accept" something if you have an awareness of it. So, in our usage, all acceptance is mindful acceptance.

Acceptance is a word that has different meanings to different people. When I refer to the skill of acceptance in this book, I'm referring to the ability to recognize what's happening in your immediate experience and choose to respond to it with openness and willingness to allow it to be as it is.

Acceptance is an alternative to fighting against your experience—trying not to feel or think something. Struggle makes your suffering worse—and does not make the problem easier.

We don't have full control over the thoughts, feelings, and physical sensations we experience, and we don't always have control over the circumstances in which we find ourselves. Taking a calm survey of your present experience and accepting how things are in this moment is a practical and useful way to respond to situations that we don't have full control over so that we don't make things worse for ourselves.

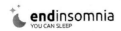

(If the term acceptance feels hard to get behind, you could also think of it as the skill of *making room* for your thoughts, feelings, sensations, and urges. When you make room for them to be there, you can find a more spacious relationship to distress, and, with practice, you will be able to tolerate difficult experiences with more groundedness and ease.)

What Acceptance Is NOT

Practicing acceptance does not mean that you are "accepting that you have insomnia and you are never going to get over it." Acceptance is about your *relationship to what is happening* in the present moment.

You don't need to sign up to accept discomfort and fatigue forever. Rather, just in this moment, can you accept what is happening in your experience and not struggle against it? Even if it is discomfort and fatigue?

Acceptance is a very practical skill that can help you break out of ingrained patterns of reactivity, respond to what's happening in empowering ways, and find a bit more ease in your situation, even if discomfort is present.

Acceptance also doesn't mean that you fixate on distressing thoughts or feelings and that you take them extremely seriously. It doesn't mean you just sit and suffer. Acceptance just means that, in the present moment, you're not resisting what is.

When you notice and accept what's happening in the present without struggling against it, then you have the choice of where you put your energy in response. From this perspective, there is a lot you can do to increase the quality of your life, suffer less, and do things that are meaningful to you—even if there are things that are difficult and that you can't control.

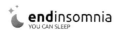
As you learn to take a more accepting attitude toward what is, poor sleep becomes less of a catastrophic event. As your insomnia experiences become less threatening, your nervous system will gradually open up to sleep.

You don't have to accept all the discomfort in your life. If there are things you can do to help yourself feel better, that's great, and you should do those things.

However, there are many times when you will experience difficult thoughts, feelings, and circumstances, and there is not much you can do about them. In those circumstances, acceptance is the best thing you can do to make your situation better. You can't control how you will sleep tonight, you don't have full control over your thoughts and feelings, and you don't have much control over the external world.

When you let go of attempting to control things that you don't have full control over, you can develop a much more peaceful relationship with whatever happens.

 NOTE:

In certain life situations outside of insomnia, such as when a person is experiencing violence or in an otherwise dangerous circumstance, the best course of action is to leave the situation. Acceptance should not be used to justify staying in an unsafe or abusive situation.

Clean vs. Dirty Pain

One key to becoming less attached to how you sleep is to reduce any unhelpful reactivity to distress that makes your experience more miserable than it needs to be. One powerful way to think about reducing unnecessary pain comes from

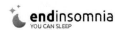

Acceptance and Commitment Therapy (ACT). Acceptance and Commitment Therapy proposes that there are two types of pain: ***clean pain*** and ***dirty pain.***

Clean pain is the unavoidable pain we feel when something difficult happens in our lives. For example, clean pain could include experiencing loss, the sadness or frustration that comes with disappointment, anxiety about the future— or fatigue from not sleeping well. Painful emotions and experiences are an inevitable part of being human.

Dirty pain, on the other hand, is the pain that arises from our subjective response to clean pain. Through the way we react, we can amplify the original pain into something much more distressing and disruptive.

Here are some common sources of dirty pain:

+ Desperately struggling against painful emotions, thoughts, and body sensations

+ Evaluating your experience in extreme or catastrophic ways

+ Never questioning the story you're telling yourself

+ Letting difficult thoughts and feelings paralyze you or keep you from doing the things that matter to you

+ Criticizing and berating yourself when you experience difficulty or pain

+ Giving in to unhelpful coping strategies that end up creating more suffering in the long run

+ Becoming so accustomed to your suffering that you have a hard time experiencing anything besides what you have come to expect

Holding the frame of clean pain vs. dirty pain in your mind is extremely helpful when working through insomnia. It invites you to consider that there is a substantial portion of your emotional distress that you have control over and can learn to reduce. Much of the suffering of people with insomnia comes from dirty pain.

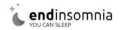

The Tug-of-War Metaphor

One helpful metaphor to practice acceptance is tug of war. Someone with insomnia is often like someone playing a brutal game of tug of war with a monster.

The Insomnia Monster is big, scary, and very strong. You stand on one side of a bottomless pit, and the Insomnia Monster stands on the other. The rope stretches across the pit, and you both pull in opposing directions. You are terrified of falling into the pit; you pull desperately on the rope.

You try to gain ground, but the harder you pull, the harder the monster pulls back. You feel yourself at the edge, so you pull even harder. You think to yourself that if you could just pull hard enough, the monster would fall into the pit, your distress would be gone, and you could finally sleep.

It would all be over, and you wouldn't feel so horrible during the day or so agonized at night. However, as hard as you try, it seems impossible to pull the monster into the pit.

This metaphor applies to both struggling at night and struggling against the distress you experience during the day.

Can you imagine how hard it would be to fall asleep while playing such a high-stakes game?

Can you imagine how hard it would be to play that game—and simultaneously engage in your life in a fulfilling and meaningful way?

So, what can you do? You can drop the rope.

You don't need to play the game. Although the monster might still be there, you don't need to fight. As you drop the rope and give up the struggle against things you can't control, you begin to suffer less; you begin to reclaim your life.

In this way, acceptance substantially lowers the stakes of getting to sleep.

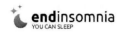

ACCEPTANCE EXERCISE:
DROPPING THE ROPE

Here's a quick exercise to get a taste of what acceptance can feel like.

To begin, take a breath and notice what's happening in your present-moment experience. (You might find it helpful to close your eyes as you do this, but you don't have to.)

Become aware of any unpleasant thoughts, feelings, or body sensations—perhaps something related to insomnia.

Take a moment to observe the difficult thought, feeling, or sensation. Notice any ways you've been struggling against its presence.

Now, bring to mind the image of tug-of-war, and see if you can feel it in your body.

Then imagine dropping the rope.

As you do so, let go of any struggle against the difficult thought, feeling, or sensation. Actually see and feel the rope dropping.

As you imagine dropping the rope, take a deep breath in. As you exhale, see if you can release any tension you are holding in your body.

Now notice any shifts toward more ease and acceptance of what is. It doesn't mean the difficult thought, feeling, or sensation is necessarily gone, just that there's more space for it to be part of your experience without needing to do anything to change it. Try to stay with this experience for the next minute.

Dropping the rope in your imagination as you've done in this exercise is a concrete way to invite your body and mind to shift from resistance to greater acceptance.

You can repeat this exercise as often as you like to help you move toward more acceptance. Doing this exercise doesn't guarantee you'll suddenly feel calm or happy—but it will allow you to experience less resistance to what is.

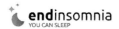

More on Mindful Acceptance

It is not enough to just think that acceptance and mindfulness are nice ideas. If you want to experience change, you need to apply them.

The skills of mindful acceptance and non-reactivity grow with practice. Maybe just reading about these ideas gives you some comfort, but the real transformation comes when you bring more mindful acceptance into your daily life.

You don't need to practice all day long, but taking moments throughout the day to consciously choose to notice and accept the present will help you begin to experience the changes you're reading about.

Especially at first, it is often unnerving to begin to relate with more acceptance toward the distressing thoughts, feelings, sensations, and circumstances that you've worked so hard to avoid. Accepting what is takes courage.

As you become more skilled at relating to your difficulties with openness and acceptance, you can train yourself over time to experience painful or challenging thoughts, feelings, and physical sensations in a way that is less threatening.

With time you will become more confident that you can handle your own mind and life in a more calm and grounded way, no matter what thoughts, feelings, or experiences come up. These changes make you more resilient to the possibility of poor sleep in the short term—and help you have a less anxious nervous system, which helps your sleep in the long term.

Less anxiety means a lower sleep-stopping force—and a higher likelihood of falling asleep and staying asleep easily.

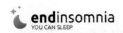

USING THE END INSOMNIA SYSTEM TO SUFFER LESS THROUGH MINDFUL ACCEPTANCE - A STORY YOU MAY RELATE TO

You may have suffered from insomnia for years before discovering the End Insomnia System. If you're like many others, your insomnia started during an intense period of stress. And then your sleep never returned to normal. Sleeping pills may have helped some, but your sleep was still very poor and inconsistent.

The worst part about your insomnia may be how bad you feel during the day. Like you're hindered and demoralized by deep fatigue, plus severe anxiety about your insomnia.

You may even suffer from so much physical depletion that you switched to part-time work or pulled back from your friendships. If you manage to maintain a romantic relationship, it's likely you feel your insomnia put a strain on it. Your life is more about surviving each day than enjoying your life...or doing the things that matter to you.

Because so much of your struggle involves how you feel during the day, a primary focus of work with the system will be learning how to suffer less during the day as a way to lower the stakes on sleep at night. To start, simply learning that your sleeping issues are driven by anxiety—and that there are steps you can take to address this—can be a huge relief.

However, the years of feeling trapped in the agony of insomnia leaves a traumatic imprint, so there's a lot of anxiety and hyperarousal to unravel. Once you've gained confidence that there is a way out of this mess, you'll start to untangle the vicious cycle of insomnia. You'll begin by implementing the sleep-window guidelines from Chapter 8 to increase your sleep-starting force. Once that's in place, you'll focus on easing your chronic worry, conditioned hyperarousal, and emotional pain.

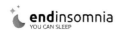

You'll come to realize that a lot of what you feel is dirty pain (subjectively amplified pain). Feeling hopeless about your insomnia for so long leads you to make catastrophic evaluations of your situation, making long nights of wakefulness and days of fatigue even more debilitating.

In that case, one of the best steps to take is to develop a daily mindfulness practice. From a place of mindful awareness, you'll practice "dropping the rope"—struggling less against how you feel and the thoughts that appear in your mind. You'll become more aware of your counterproductive thought spirals... and learn to experience poor sleep in a less threatening way.

Though insomnia may be one of the hardest things you've ever faced, you'll discover a sense of refuge in the present moment. Even when you experience worries about the night to come—or waves of fatigue during the day—you'll turn your attention to the present, and recognize, "In this moment, I'm okay."

You'll begin to feel more capable of making room for difficult thoughts and feelings that come up—without letting them dominate your experience the way they used to. This shift leads to feeling more confident that you can handle whatever happens—and overcome your insomnia.

As you become more mindfully aware and accepting of the parts of your experience that you can't control, you'll begin to find your days more bearable. As you see parts of the burden of insomnia lighten in your life, you'll develop deeper trust that you will truly be able to resolve your insomnia.

You'll begin to engage more fully with your life and tap into your values to find more meaning in your days—even when you feel bad (you'll learn how in Chapter 12).

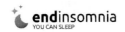

You'll reconnect with friends and push yourself outside your comfort zone through activities like taking trips or sleeping away from home. You may find yourself taking on more at work and feeling more confident professionally. You'll prioritize making the most of your days, regardless of your fatigue.

Reclaiming your days will help you become more accepting of difficult nights.

Soon, your life is no longer about insomnia, so performance anxiety around sleep begins to fade. When you don't need sleep to happen—and don't worry so much when you find yourself awake at night—your sleep-starting force will carry you into natural sleep without being impeded by the sleep-stopping force.

You'll find yourself thrilled to start sleeping more consistently than you have in months or years. As your confidence in the process continues to grow, you'll be able to wean off sleeping pills and come to trust in your natural ability to sleep without external aids.

Over about 3 to 6 months, it's likely your sleep returns to normal. Through the changes you made, you'll find that you reversed much of the anxiety and conditioned hyperarousal that used to keep you awake at night.

And through continuing the skills you learned in the End Insomnia System, you'll continue to sleep well generally—and you'll know how to resolve occasional setbacks. You'll have enough positive sleep experiences under your belt to develop a strong trust in your ability to sleep, even if a bit of anxiety is present from time to time.

Ultimately, you'll find you've learned to trust in your own power to create the conditions for natural sleep.

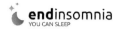
Working With Emotions

Painful emotions are one of the most difficult things to find acceptance of in the present moment. Here is an exercise to practice this important skill:

EXERCISE: MINDFUL ACCEPTANCE OF PAINFUL EMOTIONS

To bring greater mindful acceptance to painful emotions such as anxiety, sadness, frustration, and fear, here are some steps to follow:

1. Notice what emotion you are feeling and how the emotion shows up in your body. For example, do you feel tension, heat or coldness, tightness, heaviness, jitteriness, or trembling? Where in your body do you feel these things?

2. Label the emotion by saying to yourself (in your mind or aloud), "I'm feeling [insert emotion here] right now." Also, note if you are feeling multiple emotions at the same time. Psychological research shows we are better able to regulate our emotions when we can put a label on what we are feeling.

3. Allow the emotion and the corresponding body sensations to be exactly as they are. Don't force the feeling to change. Open up to it and see if you can relax any tension in your body. See if you can bring an attitude of curiosity and gentleness to your experience of the emotion. Stay with the emotion for as long as feels natural, allowing it to *be* without struggling against it.

This exercise is not intended to make your emotions go away. Rather the point is to help you acknowledge your emotions—and tolerate them with less reactivity and less dirty pain.

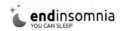

When faced with a difficult emotion like grief, anger, or strong anxiety, it is extremely helpful to remember that emotions are impermanent. When you are in the midst of a painful emotion, it can feel like it will go on forever. You might begin to assess how bleak the future looks from the standpoint of the emotion you are currently feeling.

However, emotions change. If you pay attention to your emotions, you will see for yourself that this is true. When you can open up to your emotions with less struggle, there is more space for them to flow through you and shift. Bringing acceptance to your emotions also helps to cut down on the dirty pain you might experience based on how you react to an unpleasant emotion.

Opening up to your emotions doesn't mean you just sit there and feel all day. It's important to engage in meaningful and life-enhancing activities during the day, even if a heavy emotion is present as you do so.

Just as difficult emotions are impermanent, so are miserable nights and bleary-eyed days. The journey through insomnia is full of ups and downs. So when things feel especially hard, remember: You will find a way, and things will change.

KEY CHAPTER TAKEAWAYS

+ **Mindfulness** is the skill of being intentionally aware of what's happening in the present moment without judgment.

+ **Acceptance** is the skill of opening up to your present-moment experience (your thoughts, emotions, physical sensations, or present circumstance) and allowing it to be as it is. Acceptance is an alternative to (1) trying to hide from your experience, or (2) struggling against your experience and trying to force it to change.

+ **Mindfulness and acceptance** go hand in hand.

+ Clean vs. Dirty Pain:

  ▪ **Clean pain** is the inevitable pain we experience when hard things happen in life.

  ▪ **Dirty pain** is the additional pain we experience through the ways we react to clean pain, including:

    ▸ Struggling unhelpfully against parts of our experience we don't have full control over.

    ▸ Evaluating what is happening in inaccurate or extreme ways.

    ▸ Judging ourselves harshly.

+ By becoming more mindful and accepting of your experience in the day and the night, you can decrease unnecessary suffering (dirty pain). This, in turn, helps you feel less threatened by your experience of insomnia and, with time and practice, helps your nervous system settle into a sleep-compatible state.

+ When working to accept painful emotions, remember that all emotions are impermanent. The most difficult of times will pass. Just keep going.

CHAPTER 10

Managing Anxious Thoughts

Reducing the Sleep-Stopping Force by Developing a New Relationship With Your Thoughts

In the last chapter, we talked about applying mindful acceptance to difficult emotions. Now let's turn our attention to thoughts.

Managing anxious thoughts deserves some special attention, as anxiety-filled thoughts are one of the main drivers of insomnia. It's common to experience an uptick in anxious thoughts as night approaches—and yet again in the middle of the night.

Many people with insomnia commonly report that a single thought can send them spiraling into a pit of anxiety. You may have a sense of walking on eggshells in your own mind to avoid setting off an avalanche of anxiety that makes it even harder to sleep.

How we understand and relate to our thoughts can determine the amount of dirty pain we experience related to insomnia.

There are two helpful techniques to relate to anxious thoughts—both of which rely on mindfulness (because you need to be *aware* of what you're thinking to have a new response to it):

+ **Challenge** them.

+ **Change your relationship** with them.

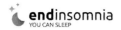

Thought Challenging

Challenging your thoughts involves (1) becoming aware of your thoughts, (2) recognizing when you have a thought that may not be grounded in reality, and (3) questioning its validity.

When you notice you are having catastrophic thoughts, it can be helpful and calming to reassure yourself by reminding yourself that your worst-case scenario fears may be inaccurate.

For example, you might find yourself in bed thinking, "I won't be able to get through tomorrow if I don't get to sleep soon." In this case, you might remind yourself of the times you've had rough nights and have still made it through the day. Even better would be to remind yourself of the times you had a rough night and got to the end of the day and realized it was not as bad as you had anticipated.

Here's another example. Let's say you have a thought such as, "If I don't sleep tonight, then I'll be too anxious to sleep the next night, and then I'm going to continue to sleep worse and worse until I never sleep at all, and then I'll die."

Thoughts like this are truly not grounded in reality.

If this kind of thought comes up, it can be helpful to remind yourself of the sleep knowledge you've gained through reading this book. In this case, you would want to remind yourself that if you have a night (or several) of rough sleep, you will have increased your sleep drive as a result (Chapter 8). Remember, a stretch of bad sleep paradoxically causes your body to force you to sleep (via your natural sleep drive) before you go too long without.

You might also remind yourself that insomnia cannot kill you (Chapter 7).

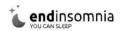

THOUGHT-CHALLENGING
EXERCISE

Here are some guidelines for challenging any thoughts that cause you distress. While following these guidelines does not guarantee that your anxiety or difficult emotions will disappear, it may help you feel better or see your situation in a more realistic and less extreme way.

1. Describe the situation that's leading to the thought.

2. What is my interpretation of the situation? This is the thought you are challenging. Look out for all-or-nothing thinking or extreme predictions.

3. What emotion(s) am I feeling that are related to this thought? What is the intensity of the emotion (1–10)?

4. **Challenge the thought:**

   a. What are other possibilities apart from my first thought?

   b. Is this thought accurate based on what I've learned about how sleep works?

   c. What's the likelihood of the worst-case scenario happening?

   d. If the worst does happen, what will I do to cope?

5. Based on this re-evaluation of the situation, does the original emotion fit? Do I feel any different emotionally now? Has the intensity (1–10) changed?

While this is a more formal procedure for challenging thoughts, it doesn't have to take this much effort. You can also **challenge thoughts in real-time** just by catching yourself having a worrisome thought and questioning if it's fully accurate based on your knowledge and past experience.

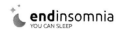

■ Limitations of Thought Challenging

Thought challenging is most helpful when your anxious thoughts are based on inaccurate assumptions about sleep. However, thought challenging will often fall short of bringing you full relief. There are two reasons for this.

First, thought challenging may help you feel a bit better, but it is not powerful enough on its own to overcome deeply conditioned hyperarousal or memories of traumatic insomnia experiences. What you need to overcome insomnia is to have the actual *experience* of feeling safe—which you can achieve through learning and applying all the tools of the End Insomnia System over time.

The second reason that thought challenging falls short is that you often can't talk yourself out of anxiety when some degree of anxiety is warranted. For example, even if you challenge a thought like, "If I don't sleep soon, I'm going to feel awful tomorrow," by reminding yourself that you've survived in the past, the fact is, tomorrow really might be a hard day.

Some people get attached to thought challenging as a way to try to ward off their anxiety and keep themselves from experiencing the outcomes they are afraid of, such as getting poor sleep. Thought challenging done with a rigid or desperate intention to force your anxiety to go away can quickly become another way you are playing an unhelpful tug-of-war with the insomnia monster.

Mindful Acceptance of Thoughts (Defusion)

So, while thought challenging can take the edge off certain thoughts, ultimately, there is a need to **accept the possibility of anxiety**. In doing so, you can gradually work to find greater resilience and feel less threatened by the possibility of poor sleep.

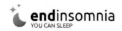

Bringing mindful acceptance to difficult thoughts serves this goal. First, it provides a way to *come to terms* with sometimes having anxious thoughts. Second, without denying the reality of the difficulty you face, mindful acceptance allows you to *cultivate a relationship* with your thoughts in which you feel less negatively affected by them and can hold them more lightly, even if you can't make them go away.

Acceptance and Commitment Therapy (ACT) offers a specific type of mindful acceptance called "defusion" to help you get space from—and perspective on—your thoughts. To be "defused" from your thoughts means the opposite of being "fused" with them (think *de-fused*.) Being fused with your thoughts is to be caught up in them—to feel as though you are your thoughts.

Through defusion techniques, you catch yourself in the act of thinking—and then step back. This allows you to become the observer of your thoughts rather *than* being your thoughts. When you can be the observer of your thoughts, you become less reactive to them and are less likely to have your actions controlled by unhelpful thoughts.

Defusion becomes more effective when we realize two important facts about thoughts:

- ✦ Fact 1: Thoughts are input, not reality.
- ✦ Fact 2: Thoughts are impermanent.

Let's break those down:

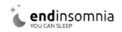

■ Fact 1: Thoughts Are Mental Input, Not Objective Reality

First, when approaching thoughts, it's helpful to frame them just as mental input instead of objective reality. We often take our thoughts extremely seriously—we feel that simply because we have a thought, it means the thought is true.

Thoughts can be incredibly useful and powerful tools, but they can also be chaotic, inaccurate, and paralyzing. Although thoughts may carry important information about our life and our environment that we should listen to, sometimes, it's not helpful to take our thoughts so seriously. It's useful to think of thoughts as "offerings" that your brain is giving you—offerings that you get to decide what to do with.

When you see your thoughts as mental input, you begin to question the authority of your thoughts—and you gain more choice about how you will respond. If you notice that a thought is giving you important guidance and is helpful, then perhaps you will let that thought inform your decision-making.

However, if you notice a thought is unhelpful or is just looping anxiously in your mind, you might choose not to take that thought as a fact you must heed. Rather than fixating on the thought, you can choose to redirect your attention to the present moment and the task at hand. Doing so doesn't necessarily mean that the unhelpful thought will immediately disappear, but it allows you to experience that thought with less reactivity and less dirty pain.

For example, you may have a thought urging you to do things that could undermine your progress through insomnia, such as making unhelpful sleep efforts or not sticking to your sleep window. If you can mindfully step back from such thoughts, you can recognize that just because you have the thought doesn't mean you must do as it says—you can choose to stay on the path toward long-term good sleep.

Additionally, from a mindful stance, you can have compassion for the part of you that is anxious without being completely consumed or controlled by that anxiety. (More to come on treating yourself compassionately in Chapter 13.)

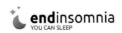
DEFUSION TOOL 1:
LABELING "THINKING"

One way to step back from your thoughts is to notice when you have a thought—and then simply say to yourself, **"Thinking."**

By labeling your experience as "thinking," you create a degree of separation between you and the thought. When you are caught in the narrative of a string of thoughts, if you can **notice** it's happening and **label** your experience, you come back into the present and can choose what you do next.

Sometimes thoughts are helpful, and you will want to give them your attention. Other times, you might notice yourself stuck in an unhelpful cycle of rumination. In the latter case, labeling your experience of "thinking" allows you to pause and change course so you don't keep mentally spinning.

As an alternative to labeling your thoughts as "thinking," you could say to yourself, "Oh, I'm having a thought" or "I'm having the thought that [fill in the blank]." Go with whatever feels most natural to you to step back and become the observer of your thoughts.

■ Fact 2: Thoughts Are Impermanent

The second premise that defusion is built upon is that thoughts are impermanent. They come and go—often very quickly. When you can step back from your thinking process and see a thought as just a thought, you can begin to hold your thoughts more lightly—and notice how they come and go. Even if you try your hardest to hold onto a thought for as long as possible, before long, you will find the thought has vanished, and you will be thinking about other things.

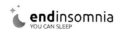

Try a thought experiment: Set a timer for five minutes and—with no goal in mind—just notice how often your thoughts change.

If you are like most of us, you might start by looking at something in the space around you...and be reminded of something that happened yesterday...which might remind you of an errand you need to run or a call you need to make... which might remind you of something else you want to do...and then a sudden sound will distract you, and then...

You get the idea. Set a timer and try this for yourself.

When you come to trust that thoughts are impermanent, you develop faith that how you view a situation will not always be the same. (For example, you might have extreme thoughts about your situation in the middle of the night but see things quite differently the next day.) With practice, it becomes easier to hold your thoughts more lightly and be less affected by the anxious ones.

While thoughts are impermanent, they can also be persistent—especially when you are in a situation that is causing you anxiety. When you use a defusion technique like labeling your thinking, it doesn't mean that you suddenly won't have that thought anymore. Such anxious thoughts might reappear again and again.

In that case, you might need to repeatedly notice these thoughts and then **redirect your attention** to the task at hand.

You can also tell yourself something like "I allow these thoughts to be present." This can give you distance from the thoughts so that you are less reactive to them.

The point of using defusion techniques is not to block out your thoughts or force them to go away. The point is to make room for your thoughts to be present without fighting them, to hold them more lightly, and to commit to doing what is important to you and what will serve your long-term journey toward great sleep—even if anxious thoughts come along for the ride.

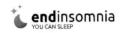

DEFUSION TOOL 2:
SINGING YOUR THOUGHTS

Another way to practice defusion and put some distance between yourself and a distressing thought is to sing it: Sing your thought to a light-hearted tune. (You could also say the thought in a silly voice.)

While this may sound a little ridiculous, that's actually the point. When you can sing a distressing thought like "If I don't take a pill soon, there's no chance I will sleep tonight," or "I can't tolerate this for another second," to the tune of a song like "Happy Birthday" or "Mary Had a Little Lamb," you will be less under the spell of this thought.

The point of this technique is not to trivialize or mock your thoughts. They might be coming from a place inside of you that is very scared, which is valid. The point of this tool is simply to help you step back from automatically buying into the thought as an absolute truth that must dictate your actions.

For example, let's say you've come off sleeping pills, but you still keep them around just in case. Then on a particularly distressing night, you are tempted to take a pill, even though you know it would be better to prove to yourself that you can survive the night without pills. If you were to sing a thought like, "If I don't take a pill soon, there's no chance I will sleep tonight," you give yourself a chance to gain a little perspective on the thought. You could recognize that although you're afraid and the idea of taking a pill is comforting, it's more important to stick to the plan of not taking a pill, even if it means facing discomfort in the short term.

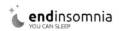

Again, using defusion techniques doesn't mean that your worries are gone or that you will not feel the discomfort of the situation that is giving rise to the thought. Rather, these techniques help you find yourself in the present moment, hold your thoughts more lightly, and have more clarity of mind to take actions that will lead you toward overcoming insomnia in the long term. We'll talk more about nighttime and daytime actions you can take to move toward long-term better sleep in Chapters 11 and 12, respectively.

Does your mind feel like a mess? Join us at the **End Insomnia Program**. We'll help you stay on track as you bring practices like mindfulness, acceptance, and defusion into your life so you can begin to relate to even the most distressing thoughts and feelings in more empowered and grounded ways.

Our community can give you support, empathy, and companionship as you make the changes described in this book. Our coaches can answer your questions and give you the accountability to make what you're learning stick. Use the link below to learn more:

https://endinsomnia.com/program

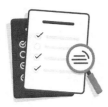

KEY CHAPTER TAKEAWAYS

☑ Thought challenging can help ease some of your anxiety when you are caught in catastrophic thinking not based on facts, but is not intended to completely wipe out your anxiety.

☑ Defusion techniques help you bring mindful acceptance to thoughts so you can:

- Get space from distressing thoughts so you are not controlled by them.

- Learn to hold your thoughts more lightly and feel less threatened by them over time.

☑ Defusion is *not* a way to force thoughts to go away.

☑ Defusion tool 1: Notice and internally label your thoughts as "thinking."

☑ Defusion tool 2: Sing a particularly distressing thought out loud to the tune of a light-hearted song, or say the thought in a silly voice.

CHAPTER

11

What to Do at Night When You Can't Get to Sleep

Calming the Sleep-Stopping Force by Softening Your Attachment to Sleep and Finding Peace When Awake

When you are awake at night and you don't want to be, there are things you can do that will make your situation worse. And there are things you can do to make your situation better—both in the moment and in service to overcoming insomnia in the long term.

Maybe your goal has been trying to sleep. Let's talk about a new goal: *Finding true peace at night, even when you can't sleep.*

In this chapter, you will learn **three helpful options** for responding to unwanted wakefulness at night. None of these options aim to force sleep to happen—that would be a sleep effort, right? You truly cannot control your sleep on a night-by-night basis.

Instead, using these options will help you gradually retrain your nervous system to be more sleep-compatible at night. Applying these three options will help you gradually dial down the sleep-stopping force (anxiety and hyperarousal) so that sleep can happen without effort.

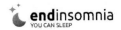

Three Options for When You're Awake at Night

You can choose:

+ Mindfulness in bed.

+ Relaxing activity in bed.

+ Relaxing activity out of bed.

Here is more on each:

■ Option 1: Mindfulness in Bed

Option one is to practice mindfulness in bed. If your nighttime default is spiraling into anxiety, a mindfulness practice can occupy your mind so that you are less caught up in worry. Ways to practice mindfulness in bed include focusing on your breath (as in Chapter 9) or doing a mindful body scan (like the exercise below).

Compared to tossing and turning and making sleep efforts, mindfully directing your awareness to your breath or body sensations may help you open to a bit more rest and relaxation, even if you also feel anxious. Learning how to face the experience of being awake with greater mindfulness can also help train your system to tolerate anxious thoughts and emotional discomfort with greater even-mindedness and less reactivity.

Practicing mindfulness in bed is no guarantee that you will fall asleep. You should not do this as a sleep effort—which won't work. To avoid the sleep-effort trap, you need to be engaging in mindfulness for its own sake. Remember:

+ Sleep efforts target a short-term goal: "Sleep NOW!" (How restful is that?)

+ Practicing mindfulness is a long-term investment in overcoming your insomnia—and, ironically, when practiced for its own sake (and not as a sleep effort), it can also have immediate short-term calming effects.

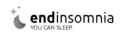

Of course, you would rather be sleeping than practicing mindfulness in the middle of the night. However, see if you can come to view wakefulness as an opportunity to practice developing your mindfulness skills for the sake of personal growth and to support your journey toward long-term improved sleep. If you can do so, you will be able to experience being awake as at least a bit more acceptable.

(To boost your incentive to practice mindfulness for its own sake, check out Chapter 14, which takes a deeper dive into the benefits of and science behind mindfulness —specifically, mindfulness meditation.)

MINDFULNESS EXERCISE: BODY SCAN

A body scan is a mindfulness exercise in which you "scan" your attention through your body, starting with your toes and working up your legs and torso, through your arms, and to the top of your head. You can choose how fast to scan through the different parts of your body— very slowly or relatively quickly. To start, you might try spending about 15 seconds on each body part. The point is just to *mindfully observe* the sensations in each body part without trying to change them.

Start with your toes and put all your awareness into just the sensations you feel in your toes for 15 seconds. Then move on to feeling the sensations in your feet, and then keep moving up through your body, spending roughly 15 seconds in each body part.

Here is a sequence you can follow in your body scan:

+ Toes
+ Feet
+ Ankles
+ Lower legs

+ Knees
+ Upper legs
+ Pelvis
+ Lower torso

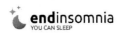
- Chest
- Upper back
- Hands
- Lower arms
- Elbows

- Upper arms
- Neck
- Back of your head
- Face
- Top of your head

When you get to the top of your head, you can scan down your body again in the reverse direction. Do this as long as you like, finding a pace that feels right to you.

Again, you're welcome to spend more than 15 seconds on each body part. You don't even have to count; just spend a while on each body part before moving to the next.

When you notice that your mind is wandering or that you've become distracted, return your attention to where you left off and continue scanning through your body. If you find that you can't feel anything in a particular body part, just notice the absence of feeling, and then carry on with your body scan.

Some find this exercise to be soothing and pleasantly distracting as they lie in bed at night, helping them feel at least a bit more at peace with being awake, even if anxiety is also present. One beautiful thing about this exercise is that it can help you become aware of what it's like to inhabit your own body in a way you may never have experienced before. You may also feel some new appreciation for your body by becoming more aware of the subtle sensations always happening inside of you.

A body scan is also a very relaxing and grounding mindfulness exercise to practice during the day as a meditation. If you practice this during the day, you can do it sitting up or lying down.

Don't expect practicing mindfulness in bed to immediately lead to calm acceptance of being awake. However, you can gradually learn to experience less dirty pain (unnecessary suffering) at night and gain more confidence that

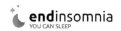

you can get through your day no matter how the night goes. Mindfulness helps train your body and mind to be less reactive.

Additionally, you may find it especially hard to maintain mindful awareness at night. If your mind wanders while in a restful state, that's okay. Normal sleepers often lie in bed resting when they can't sleep, and this is fine for you to do as well. However, if you notice yourself caught in worry and agitation, redirecting your focus to mindfulness will help.

While it's worth giving mindfulness in bed a try, it's not the best option for everyone. Option 2 or 3 may be more useful if you find it difficult to practice mindfulness in bed.

■ Option 2: Pleasant Activity in Bed

Option two is to do something you enjoy and find somewhat relaxing as you lie in bed when you can't sleep. You could read, listen to a podcast or audiobook, or watch something.

As you know, you can't force yourself to sleep. The idea here is to occupy your mind: to shift it from its tendency to fixate on worry at night and to turn being awake into at least a slightly more positive experience.

Avoid screens if you find them overstimulating. However, some find watching something to be the best way to find more acceptance and enjoyment in being awake, which helps them lower the sleep-stopping force. Finding ways that work for you to lower sleep anxiety matters much more than avoiding blue light.

You are still likely to experience some anxiety as you do your activity in bed, but occupying your attention in this way can help soothe some of the discomfort and help you find greater acceptance of being awake.

As you do your chosen activity in bed, notice when you begin to experience signs of sleepiness like your eyes getting heavy, yawning, or nodding off. At this point, stop your activity and close your eyes; see if sleep is ready to happen.

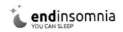

If it's not, then you're welcome to do one of these activities again or practice some mindfulness in bed. You have to be patient if sleep is not happening and allow it to **happen on its own time.** Remember: Trying to force sleep to happen will only make you more agitated and frustrated, and push sleep further away.

There will be nights where you feel more accepting and nights where you feel much less accepting—and perhaps worry you have lost all your progress. That's normal. You just have to keep going and trust the process.

■ Option 3: Pleasant Activity Out of Bed

Finally, option three is to do something pleasant and relaxing outside of bed. If your nervous system is highly agitated and you feel very stressed lying in bed, then getting out of bed for a while can be a way to give your nervous system a little reset. You may still feel agitated outside of bed, but the change of position and scene physically acts as a reboot.

When you leave your bed, even just to use the toilet, the physical change offers fresh input: it helps interrupt any subtle loops of anxiety you might have been caught in without realizing it.

To make the most of that natural shift in perspective, once you leave your bed, do something relaxing that you might enjoy. Read, listen to something, watch a show or video, or do something else you find pleasant.

When you notice you are getting sleepy (drooping eyes, yawning, or nodding off) or you've had enough, then return to bed and see if sleep is ready to happen. If you still find yourself awake some time later, you can choose to leave bed again or use one of the other two options for making peace with being awake.

Be careful here. Getting out of bed is not intended to be a calculated maneuver to make sleep happen. That would be a sleep effort, right? And sleep efforts don't work. If you choose to leave your bed, let your intention be to see if it helps you find a little bit more acceptance of being awake, even though you'd prefer to be asleep.

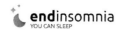

Refining the Three Options

Remember, it's not enough to just use one of the options above and hope that will be enough to make you totally calm at night. To truly feel calm at night, you must reduce anxiety across the board and become less afraid of the daytime consequences of insomnia, too. If you're extremely anxious about what will happen if you don't sleep, your progress in making peace with being awake at night will be slow.

As you combine a strategy to help you find greater acceptance at night with the other parts of this system to reduce sleep anxiety and cultivate resilience, you will gradually **retrain your nervous system** to be more **sleep-compatible** at night.

The following refinements are important to practice along with any of the three options:

+ Give up clock-watching.
+ Let go of expectations.
+ Make room for discomfort.
+ Conserve your energy.
+ Manage hyperarousal symptoms.

Let's examine these refinements in greater detail:

■ Give Up Clock-Watching

When you can't sleep, you might be in the habit of checking the clock throughout the night. Perhaps you want to monitor how the night is going, how long you slept, how long until morning, or if it's time to take additional pills or try some other sleep effort. While looking at the clock might occasionally bring some relief or a pleasant surprise, the vast majority of the time, it brings on more

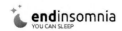

anxiety. The more you monitor the time, the more you will tend to become agitated. Analyzing and fretting over what the rest of the night or the day to come will be like just pushes sleep further away.

As I mentioned in Chapter 8, at the start of your nightly wind-down, set your alarm—and then stop looking at the clock.

This helps you to be less fixated on what time it might be and what that means for your night. When you're in bed, allow yourself to be open to sleep when it happens—without evaluating your performance via clock-watching.

If you are used to monitoring the clock, it may be uncomfortable at first to let this habit go—but as you adjust, you'll find your experience is better without clock-fueled hits of anxiety.

■ Let Go of Expectations

Let go of predictions about how you will sleep. You may be used to approaching the night with dread or hope—but you can't really know how the night will go.

Even if you have assumptions ("beliefs") based on past experience, there are no guarantees, so it's worth keeping an open mind.

Predictions and expectations cause more anxiety: Practicing acceptance of whatever comes helps you get out of your own way.

Many find this a particularly difficult habit to break—we can all get stubborn about the stories we tell ourselves. So let's explore a few examples of common beliefs people struggling with insomnia hold:

Beliefs about cycles: Someone with insomnia might have internalized an idea such as, "If I'm not asleep by a certain time, then I missed my chance—I will get a second wind, and my body won't let me sleep after that."

There's no biological rule that once a certain time—or amount of time—passes, you can't fall asleep anymore. Ideas like this are not rules: they are **self-fulfilling prophecies** fueled by anxiety and hyperarousal. Holding a false belief like this—

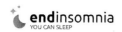

even if based on past experience—**reinforces** the false idea and creates the stress that causes it to come true.

Beliefs about patterns: You might have developed expectations about the pattern your sleep follows over several nights. This is thinking such as: "I know how my body works: I get a good night's sleep and then two bad nights after. Then a good night again, and two bad nights. Like clockwork."

It's common to feel like your body is trapped in a certain sleep pattern—but this is really another form of self-fulfilling prophecy. When you expect a poor night and feel anxious about it happening, that increases the chances that it will. Then the next night, when your sleep drive is higher, you also are less anxious because you *expect* a better night—which makes it easier for you to sleep.

Ultimately, your body is not set on any pattern of sleep. When you practice techniques to ease your sleep anxiety over time, these patterns fade.

In the meantime, do your best to keep an open mind about how the night might go and avoid self-fulling prophecies. Take comfort in knowing that there is nothing wrong with your body and that by applying the principles in the End Insomnia System, you are taking steps to address the underlying issue of sleep anxiety. Be patient in the meantime.

■ Make Room for Discomfort

As you apply any of the three options for making peace with wakefulness, it's important to expect and make room for discomfort. After all, it's not easy to be awake at night when you'd like to be asleep.

You will likely come up against a good deal of anxiety and hyperarousal at night, especially in the early stages of working through insomnia. There's no easy escape from this. The more you can preemptively be ready for discomfort, the easier it is to face it in the moment.

You are not always going to tolerate discomfort well, which is normal—and okay. But holding the intention to accept discomfort is important. Over time, you will become better at tolerating discomfort and experience it less.

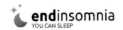

■ Conserve Your Energy

When you spend much of the night caught in reactivity and emotional distress, you expend a lot of energy. Such ragged nights can leave you feeling an extra layer of exhaustion the next day.

As you learn to make greater peace with being awake at night and become more able to access an accepting and restful state, you save a lot of energy that can help you feel better the next day.

Let's say you're someone who feels best with seven or eight hours of sleep, but because of insomnia you only get four or five hours. After a night full of struggle and anguish, four or five hours of sleep may often leave you feeling quite miserable the next day. However, as you learn to struggle less when you can't sleep and begin to feel calmer at night, you'll be surprised to find yourself feeling better than expected after a night of reduced sleep.

Don't expect to get here immediately; it takes time and practice. However, you can learn to conserve your energy at night and energize your days. And with more bearable days, your sleep "performance anxiety" will decrease, which will also help you break the insomnia cycle.

The first step of conserving energy at night is to become less reactive to the hyperarousal you experience from not sleeping. Although it's taxing to experience hyperarousal at night, it's even more taxing when your reaction to hyperarousal creates *further* hyperarousal.

The second step of conserving energy, and usually one that comes a bit later in the process of overcoming insomnia, is to begin to actually feel less hyperarousal at night. As you continue to practice the End Insomnia System, you will lower your sleep anxiety and begin to feel more at ease and calm at night. You will then naturally conserve even more energy. At this point, you're also much more likely to fall asleep and stay asleep—but even if you find yourself awake, it's much less of a big deal.

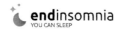

■ Manage Hyperarousal Symptoms at Night

It's common for people with insomnia to experience "inexplicable" physical symptoms at night, such as:

+ Hypnic jerks (the twitches in your body that wake you up just as you're falling asleep).
+ Drifting in and out of light sleep without seeming to enter into deeper sleep.
+ A racing heart as you lie in bed and begin to feel anxious about whether or not you will sleep.
+ Waking up in a state of alarm in the middle of the night.
+ Increasing tension in your body as you lie in bed.

Is any of that familiar? Have you wondered if these symptoms mean there is something wrong with your body or brain? Rest assured: The nervous system in hyperarousal can do all of these things and more.

These symptoms of hyperarousal are brought on by sleep anxiety. You have limited control over these symptoms when they happen, but your *reaction* to them determines whether they become worse or whether you reduce them over time.

Recognize: When you react to these experiences with alarm, that merely reinforces the sense of threat (fight-or-flight) that causes these symptoms in the first place. Demystifying these symptoms—that is, recognizing them as signs of hyperarousal—is the first step toward breaking the vicious cycle.

Accept: Next, you need to learn to become more accepting when these experiences occur. They are unpleasant and annoying, but if you can accept that they are happening and that you don't have immediate control over them, you begin to signal to your body and mind that you are safe and that no threat is present—that you don't need to be in fight-or-flight mode (i.e., hyperarousal).

Acceptance gives you the best chance of falling asleep. These symptoms fade as you lower your sleep anxiety and recondition your nervous system to be more

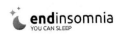

at peace at night. As you work toward that end, do your best to be patient and tolerant when you have these hyperarousal experiences, and trust that they will pass in time.

USING THE END INSOMNIA SYSTEM TO OVERCOME NIGHTTIME PANIC - A STORY YOU MAY RELATE TO

You may have been suffering from insomnia for over a year or even longer. Even if you were a good sleeper all your life, you now struggle for hours to sleep most nights. You likely read a lot of scary online articles about sleep deprivation... and your insomnia grew worse and worse.

You may find the most excruciating part of insomnia is lying awake at night. Your fear of poor sleep and the possible long-term effects it could have make facing nighttime wakefulness very difficult. Each miserable minute that ticks by feels like a confirmation of fears that you're broken and that your insomnia will slowly ruin your life. You may feel desperately alone and broken.

As you learn that anxiety is the underlying cause of your sleep issues—and that there is a way out—you'll begin to feel more grounded. The system will address your distress at night by strategizing how to find more peace when you can't sleep.

You may plan to practice mindfulness in bed, knowing it can help you feel a bit more accepting while awake. And, because you see the value of practicing mindfulness for its own sake. You'll also realize that sticking to a reasonable sleep window will give you a solid sleep drive (or sleep-starting force) when bedtime arrives.

For several weeks, you'll encounter ups and downs. You'll try to apply the plan at night, but when you get into bed and feel the fear start to grip you, ou may revert to panic... and make desperate attempts to make yourself sleep

Remember, overnight results aren't the goal of the system - it's a good start if you can find just 10-20% more peace at night.

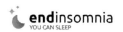

You'll find that realistic expectations help you avoid feeling like a failure or giving up when you encounter resistance or intense hyperarousal symptoms.

With time, you'll internalize that you truly can't control your sleep at night and that your best option is to find a way to be more okay with being awake. You'll also recognize that you need to willingly face your fears of having a bad night and prove to yourself that you can get through the next day regardless.

As these realizations sink in, you'll find yourself giving up your old sleep efforts and able to face the difficult feelings you encounter in the night with less reactivity and more acceptance. While this won't immediately make your nights totally peaceful, it will significantly cut down on the dirty pain you experience at night.

You'll realize that while becoming more accepting of being awake is a big step in the right direction, you also need to make the consequences of poor sleep less frightening (as in Chapter 12) before you truly feel at ease at night.

As you come to feel less affected during the day and more accepting when awake at night, you'll develop much more ease and calm. You'll feel significantly less threatened by your insomnia and develop a strong confidence that you will overcome insomnia. With greater calmness at night, you'll begin to sleep more consistently.

It'll likely take a couple of months for your unconscious mind (the part responsible for conditioned hyperarousal) to catch up to your new conscious experience.

However, you'll find yourself patient through the ups and downs in the process... and returning to normal sleep in time.

Though you still won't enjoy rough nights when they occasionally happen, you'll no longer experience them as deeply threatening. For this reason, you'll sleep better and find you're no longer plagued by worries about insomnia returning. Ultimately, you'll find the vicious cycle of insomnia has been permanently broken.

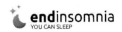

Remember That You Can't Force Sleep to Happen

Although you've heard it many times in this book already, it's crucial to remember that there is nothing you can do to force sleep to happen. Simply reminding yourself of this fact as you lie in bed can help to soften the automatic impulse to try to make yourself sleep. With time and experience, you will internalize this truth and experience the relief of knowing you don't need to work so hard. Instead of making sleep efforts, it will become second nature for you to focus on making the most of the fact that you're awake right now, knowing that's just how things are.

■ What to Remember About Sleep Stages and Cycles

Although we talked about sleep stages and sleep cycles in Chapter 3, it's worth reiterating the key takeaways that can help put your mind more at ease at night:

1. **WAKING IN THE MIDDLE OF THE NIGHT IS NORMAL.**

    At the end of each sleep cycle, it's normal to have a brief awakening, and these awakenings happen more often in the latter part of the night when sleep is lighter. When normal sleepers experience these awakenings, they usually quickly return to sleep, often without noticing the break. When you have insomnia, you may have more trouble.

    When you experience these normal awakenings, rather than quickly re-entering sleep, you might start to become conscious of—and anxious about—being awake.

    The way to deal with nighttime awakenings is to normalize them. Remind yourself it's normal and natural to wake up at night. It doesn't need to cause panic. With time, as you become more accepting of when you are awake and feel less threatened by insomnia, you will come to experience these awakenings without a strong reaction and will be able to re-enter sleep like a normal sleeper.

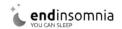

2. **THE DEEPEST REST COMES DURING THE FIRST PART OF YOUR SLEEP.**

    You experience the deepest rest and get the most restorative benefits during the first two sleep cycles. So if you get at least a few hours of sleep, you've likely gotten most if not all of your deep sleep.

    If you're able to stay awake through the day and get by, that's a sign that you're likely at least getting your "core sleep," the minimum your body can function on (even if you would function better on more sleep). How much core sleep a person needs to function varies from about 3–5 hours.

Additionally, remember that research has shown that people with insomnia often:

+   Underestimate the amount of sleep they get.

+   Perceive that they've been awake and that they did not sleep, even if laboratory equipment shows that for parts of the period in question, they were actually sleeping.

Remembering these facts about nighttime awakenings and core sleep can help you feel less alarmed about your sleep.

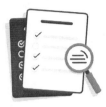

KEY CHAPTER TAKEAWAYS

☑ **Use one of these three options** at night when you can't sleep (to feel less threatened by being awake, not to make you sleep):

1. **Practice mindfulness in bed.** This is a way to find more acceptance for being awake and shift your mind from engaging in its default of unchecked worry.

2. **Do something pleasant in bed.** This is a way to occupy your mind and find more peace when you are awake. When you feel sleepy, stop the activity and see if sleep is ready to happen.

3. **Do something pleasant outside of bed.** If you feel highly anxious in bed and need a break, leave your bed and do something relaxing to help you find more peace with being awake. When you feel sleepy, return to bed and see if sleep is ready to happen.

☑ What to do along with any of the three options:

- Don't look at the clock at night. Clock-watching increases anxiety— and the sleep-stopping force.

- Let go of predictions about how the night will go.
- Expect and make room for some discomfort.
- Conserve your energy by working to make peace with being awake.
- Accept any hyperarousal symptoms, such as involuntary jerks. Symptoms of hyperarousal fade as you learn to reduce hyperarousal.

☑ Remind yourself that there is nothing you can do to force sleep to happen. The best thing you can do is work to make being awake more acceptable.

☑ It's normal to wake up multiple times during the night. As you calm your nervous system over time, you will fall back asleep like a normal sleeper.

☑ If you are able to stay awake through the day and get by, you are likely getting the core sleep your body needs.

CHAPTER

12

Finding Daytime Resilience When Fatigued

Reducing the Sleep-Stopping Force Through Lowering the Stakes on Sleep—by Living Fully

The daytime consequences of insomnia can be rough. When you get up in a state of exhaustion and are plagued during the day by fatigue and dread about the bad nights ahead, it's common to begin to pull back from doing things in your life that are important to you.

Here are some common life changes and sacrifices people with insomnia make:

+ Pull back from loved ones and social events
+ Avoid traveling
+ Cut down or quit working
+ End a romantic relationship or stop looking for one
+ Move—solely to be somewhere you think it will be easier to sleep
+ Abstain from moderate caffeine or alcohol
+ Give up hobbies, regular exercise, or other activities that used to bring you joy or fulfillment

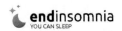

The Importance of Reengaging With Your Life

A desire to withdraw is understandable. You're struggling to sleep, you're fatigued much of the time, and you may often feel that you're living a miserable existence.

In this state, it's hard to have the will or enthusiasm to do the things that used to be important to you. You might even find it painful to do those things because you're reminded of how different things used to be. You may also be afraid of failure, worse sleep, or other painful outcomes if you try to engage in the things you used to do.

Unfortunately, when you withdraw from your life in these understandable ways, you end up focusing even more on your sleep—which makes your sleep anxiety worse.

When your life is on pause and you are not living in a fulfilling way, you will not be satisfied with your life, making the stakes on getting sleep even higher. So pulling back from your life to try to fix your insomnia—or because you just feel like you can't handle your life—actually makes the problem worse.

This is why it's so important to begin to re-engage more fully with your life— to reclaim the activities and aspirations that insomnia took from you. As you do so—and prove to yourself that you are capable of living your life fully—you will lower the stakes on sleep and take a huge step toward putting insomnia behind you.

This chapter will provide a framework to live well and do what matters to you, even when dealing with fatigue and discomfort.

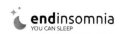

CAFFEINE AND ALCOHOL WHILE
WORKING THROUGH INSOMNIA

Abstaining from caffeine and alcohol is a common feature of many insomnia protocols. However, it's okay to have these in moderation as you work through your insomnia. Totally giving up caffeine or alcohol, if you enjoy these, can make the burden of insomnia feel even greater.

Here are guidelines that can help you bring caffeine and alcohol back if you've given them up because of insomnia:

Caffeine: For many people, having morning caffeine increases their quality of life and can help get their day on track if they feel groggy or tired in the morning. If you enjoy caffeine, it's generally fine to have some in the morning. It will not hinder your progress in working through insomnia. Your body will metabolize the caffeine in time for it not to have an impact on your sleep.

However, if you know you're especially sensitive to caffeine, be mindful not to overdo consumption (even in the morning) to avoid being wired from caffeine into the late evening. Even if you are not particularly sensitive, it is a good idea to avoid consuming it past noon (at least as you are still working through insomnia).

Alcohol: It's usually okay to have some alcohol socially if you enjoy it.

However, if you notice that alcohol significantly disrupts your sleep, which it does for some people, then as you use the End Insomnia System, it's a good idea to keep your drinking on the lighter side. If you are sensitive, avoiding or taking it easy on alcohol will help you sleep better more often, which will help you build sleep confidence.

As you get deeper into your journey through insomnia, you will care less about possible sleep disruption, and you may find you are less sensitive to alcohol's effect on your sleep. With time, you can reclaim whatever relationship you had with alcohol pre-insomnia.

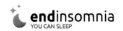

Revising the Story You Tell About Your Suffering

One of the foundational ideas of Acceptance and Commitment Therapy—and a core tenet of Buddhist philosophy for over 2500 years—is the idea that *hardship and suffering are inevitable* experiences in life.

We live in a difficult world full of uncertainty. Emotional pain, distressing thoughts, discomfort, and loss are normal parts of life. The things we're most attached to are impermanent—including our own lives. We will certainly have times when we are disappointed, hurt, or even devastated by circumstances or by the people around us. Things don't always go the way we want.

That's not to deny that life also holds great joy, beauty, and wonder. It does. But encountering suffering is inevitable; it's part of being human.

This goes against a lot of cultural messaging that says if we're not constantly happy and thriving, something is terribly wrong and we need to fix it. This is a message perpetuated by social media, where people create very well-crafted representations of their lives—manipulated versions that edit out the turmoil they might also be experiencing or the parts of their lives that aren't so polished.

Advertising also leverages the message that if we're not feeling great or achieving some standard, there's something wrong with us. We're told we should buy this car, these clothes, or whatever other product to fix ourselves.

When you accept that sometimes life is inevitably hard, you can stop beating yourself up for having a hard time (which only makes you feel worse). When you stop pathologizing yourself for experiencing difficulty, you can find a way to move forward with your life—you become more resilient in the face of adversity because you expect it.

Additionally, when you accept the difficulty of life, you can choose to do things that are meaningful enough to you to make the challenges of life worth facing. Identifying and living out your values is one powerful way to meet the challenges of life with greater resilience and to find meaning even in the midst of adversity.

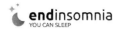

Connecting With Your Values

Values are qualities that you can live out on a daily basis through your actions. They are ways of being that you prioritize, and that bring meaning and fulfillment to your life. Some examples of common values are honesty, community, justice, rationality, love, health, humor, kindness, learning, and spirituality.

Acting upon your values is inherently meaningful, not specifically because it yields positive outcomes (though it may), but rather because it feels good to live your life in accordance with your beliefs and priorities. Living out your values can give your life a sense of purpose despite any difficulty that may be present.

■ The Risks of Losing Touch With Your Values in Pursuit of Goals

Values are different from goals. Goals are definite outcomes that you hope to achieve and that can be checked off. In contrast, values are qualities that you can act on in the present moment that bring meaning to you as you engage with them.

You can complete goals; you can never "complete" your values. Values are ways of being and doing that you can always tap into. In this way, they provide a lasting source of meaning.

Let's further examine the divide between goals and values to make a strong case for becoming more conscious of your personal values.

Goals are very important. They can give us a great sense of purpose and motivation. It's natural to want to achieve or acquire certain things and to put energy into going after them.

However, goals are not a wise thing to build our entire sense of life purpose around. First, this is because we may not achieve our goals. We may have goals that are unrealistic and beyond our capacity to achieve. Or perhaps, despite our

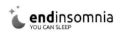

best efforts, something gets in the way. Building your entire sense of purpose around something that you may or may not achieve is a recipe for disappointment.

The second issue with over-centering goals in our lives is that even if we achieve our goals, we have likely overestimated the fulfillment that reaching the goal will bring. There is a researched-support idea in psychology called hedonic adaptation (from Greek hēdonikos "pleasurable"). It is also known as the "hedonic treadmill."

Here's how hedonic adaptation works: First, we have a baseline level of happiness in our lives. We believe we will be significantly happier in a lasting way once we achieve some goal in the future. However, once we achieve the goal, though we experience a temporary spike in our happiness, we eventually return to the baseline happiness we had before attaining the goal. We become used to the new thing in our lives, and it stops feeling so special.

At this point, we tend to look for a new "new thing" to go after in life that we hope will bring us truly lasting happiness. We stay on the **hedonic treadmill,** seeking greater happiness but ultimately staying at about the same happiness level.

Hedonic adaptation was initially demonstrated in a classic 1978 research paper that examined the happiness of lottery winners and people who were paralyzed as a result of an accident.

The study found that, after a few months, lottery winners were not happier than a control group who did not win the lottery. Additionally, the people who became paralyzed were not substantially less happy than non-disabled people once they adjusted to the initial change.

Since then, many more studies have supported the idea that whether an event is good or bad, in most cases, we adapt to what has happened and find our baseline again, often relatively quickly.

Think back on times in your own life when you might have thought, "Once I have this *[relationship/house/job/degree/vacation/salary/whatever]*, then everything will be different, and I'll really be happy." You may recognize that

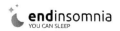

once you got the thing you were seeking, at some point, it just became a normal part of your life, and you returned to a baseline level of life satisfaction.

Some things we achieve in life can bring lasting changes in our general happiness and well-being—if they help us meet our basic needs for things like security, safety, connection, and belonging. However, generally speaking, the bump in happiness we experience when we reach our goals eventually wears off.

Does this mean we're doomed to always feel the way we do now? Fortunately, no. Checking off goals may not bring lasting happiness, but it doesn't mean there are no ways to increase your level of overall happiness and satisfaction in life.

Sonja Lyubomirsky, a positive psychologist and researcher, draws on a range of happiness research to back her proposition that three primary factors are responsible for happiness:

1. **Our genetic happiness set point** (this is the genetic influence on your baseline happiness level).
2. **Our life circumstances** (money, the state of our health, how conventionally attractive we are, job, family situation, etc.).
3. **The intentional activities** we choose to engage in.

Lyubomirsky asserts that, due to hedonic adaptation, **our happiness is determined substantially more by our actions and choices than by the external circumstances of our lives**.

This means that what we do on a daily basis—and the mindset we bring to it—matters. This third category—our intentional activities—is where we have the most leverage to increase the quality of our life, even in the midst of challenging circumstances.

One of the most effective ways to influence our well-being is to live out our values on a daily basis. That way, we can find meaning and fulfillment in the present—rather than hoping we may finally feel fulfilled at some future point.

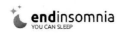

Goals are motivating and can bring with them good outcomes, but values are a way to make the journey toward the goals meaningful in and of itself.

So, when you live out your values, you're acting in inherently rewarding ways—because you are acting in alignment with the person you want to be. Doing so helps you find the resilience to weather the storms of life and keep moving forward toward what matters to you, even if you encounter painful thoughts or emotions. Even in the hardest of times (and insomnia has many hard times), your values are always available to give you a sense of meaning.

VALUES EXERCISE 1:
IDENTIFYING YOUR VALUES

Below are a few questions to ask yourself to get a sense of what your values are. Write down your answers.

+ What do you want your life to stand for?

+ How do you want to live your life?

+ At your funeral someday, what would you want someone who knows you well to say about the principles by which you lived?

There are countless values. You should connect with those values that inherently matter to you, not values that you feel you "should" have.

As you consider values that you want to live out more fully, it's best to just pick 3–5 to focus on. If you try to track more than that, it's easy to lose focus, and the meaning of your values will be diluted because there are so many you're trying to incorporate into your life.

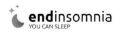

VALUES EXERCISE 2:
CREATING ACTION DEFINITIONS FOR YOUR VALUES

Again, values are ways of being in the present moment. Identifying values that resonate with you is nice—but it is only through taking action on your values and prioritizing them that they can bring you resilience and fulfillment.

For the 3–5 values you've chosen to focus on, write down an action definition for each (see some examples below). This will help you specify what acting out this value will look like. For example:

Value + Action Definition

Love: Choosing to act in loving ways toward yourself and others.

Courage: Choosing to face your fears in order to do what's important to you. Honesty: Choosing to tell the truth to others and/or to be honest with yourself.

Determination: Doing what needs to be done in a consistent way, and staying the course in the face of hardship.

Mindfulness: Finding times during your day to notice yourself in the present moment and to let your experience be exactly as it is without judgment or struggle.

Spirituality: Prioritizing time in spiritual practice, with a spiritual community, or studying your chosen spirituality.

Kindness: Choosing to be kind toward others and yourself on a daily basis.

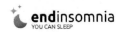

Applying Values to Your Journey Through Insomnia

Let's apply the idea of living out your values more specifically to your struggles with sleep. In order to overcome sleep anxiety, you need to (1) find more peace and acceptance when you are awake at night, and (2) make the daytime consequences of poor sleep more manageable. When both the night and daytime experiences related to insomnia are less distressing, you will have less sleep anxiety.

The last chapter focused on how to help yourself at night. As for lessening the fear of the daytime consequences of insomnia, the best thing you can do is prove to yourself that your day can be tolerable even after poor sleep—and that you can live a full life again, even before your insomnia is gone.

Combining the skills of mindfulness and acceptance with a *focus on living out your values* is a powerful way to move toward this end.

As you go through your day, you might face worrisome thoughts, emotional pain, and the physical challenges of fatigue. However, when you accept that these are part of your experience right now, and take steps to do the things that matter to you anyway, you may be surprised at how your experience changes.

Making plans to do valued activities and then following through with them is called **"behavioral activation"** in psychology. Behavioral activation is a core intervention in behavioral therapies such as CBT and ACT because a wide range of studies support it as an effective way to create shifts in mood.

Living by your values creates greater resilience, increases your tolerance for facing difficulty, and helps you have more positive experiences during the day, even if you haven't slept well.

When you are doing things that matter to you and living a full life, many times you will get to the end of the day after a rough night and realize that it was

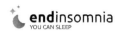

actually not as bad as you had thought it was going to be. Maybe it was a good day after all.

Having experiences like this helps you be less afraid of poor sleep in the future.

There may be times when you need to take it easy if you feel highly fatigued, but generally, it's important to try your best to live your life fully, the way you would if you didn't have insomnia. In doing so, you lower the stakes on sleep by reclaiming the life that insomnia took from you—and by proving that you are capable of having a good day after a hard night.

Along with living out your values, it can be helpful to prioritize doing some things that you simply *enjoy*. Doing activities that connect you, even briefly, with feelings of contentment or joy can help make the consequences of poor sleep feel less heavy.

USING THE END INSOMNIA SYSTEM TO DISCOVER YOUR RESILIENCE – A STORY YOU MAY RELATE TO IF YOU'RE CAREER DRIVEN

You may have been struggling with insomnia for several years. Sometimes you lay awake for hours trying to get to sleep. Other times, you may wake in the middle of the night with your heart pounding and your nervous system on edge.

You often drift between being awake and sleeping lightly for much of the night, and it's frustrating with how difficult it seems to sleep deeply. You may have even tried CBT-I, but your results weren't lasting, so you decided to try the End Insomnia System.

Like many others, the worst part of your insomnia may be how hobbled you feel in your profession. Whether you own a business or focus on your career, you have many tasks that require energy and concentration. After a bad night, you feel that your brain doesn't work well enough to stay on top of things.

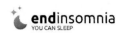

At this point, you may even split your tasks into two to-do lists. The first holds your demanding tasks, which you'll only do if you sleep decently. The second list is full of simple tasks that you'll do if you slept poorly. Yet you find yourself rarely able to get to the important things on your "slept well" list, and it's frustrating that you're limited in this way. You worry about how your career or business will be affected by having your daily schedule so determined by how you slept the night before.

Work means a lot to you. Through the system, you'll prove to yourself that you can still do demanding tasks with less sleep, and you'll begin to feel less anxious about the night. The system challenges you to connect with your values of achievement and determination—no matter how you're feeling, or what your thoughts are telling you about how incapable you are when you have little sleep.

So you'll begin to take on tasks from your hard-to-do list, no matter how you sleep. You'll treat it like a game that could lead to better sleep: If you can find a way to get things done that you didn't think you were capable of on poor sleep, you'll feel less anxious about the consequences of poor sleep and you'll have a calmer nervous system at night.

You'll begin to see that fatigued days also hold an opportunity to work through your fears and doubts (more on this in Chapter 15).

Within several weeks, you'll find you've proven to yourself that you're more capable than you thought when running on poor sleep. Although you'll still struggle with fatigue and don't feel as sharp, you'll recognize that you can still do what you need to get done without feeling professionally stunted by insomnia.

As you combine this newfound confidence with the other tools in this system to lower your sleep-stopping force, you'll gradually begin to sleep better. Within several months, you'll sleep much more consistently. And you'll find your career or business thriving again.

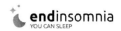

Don't Always Believe Your Mood and Energy Forecasts

When you feel especially groggy in the morning after a bad night, you will likely feel a shift as you go about your day. The same goes for a low point of energy during the day—you will likely get a second wind at some point and feel a bit better, even if you still are dealing with anxiety or background fatigue.

So be careful about making extreme predictions about how bad your day will be based on how you feel at the moment. Energy naturally fluctuates throughout the day. Even people with normal sleep often experience an afternoon slump— which can be easy to forget if you've had insomnia for a long time.

■ Overcoming Special Event Insomnia

Special event insomnia is when your anticipation of a special event the next day causes increased sleep anxiety the night before. The special event is usually something important to you, such as travel, a big day at work, a social gathering, seeing family, or something else out of the ordinary. These events create a lot of sleep anticipation because, understandably, you don't want to feel extremely tired or "off" for the event.

The hard truth is that there is no way to ensure you sleep well before a special event. Because of increased sleep anxiety before a special event, you may well have extra difficulty sleeping.

The good news is that you can resolve special event insomnia over time. The way to do this is to go through with the special event regardless of how you sleep. You must show yourself that you have the resilience to make it through and have it go well. The knowledge and skills of the End Insomnia System can make this possible for you. Face the day with acceptance and willingness to show up and do the best you can.

Once you prove to yourself that you can get through—and even have some positive moments—you'll be less afraid of it happening the next time. You'll

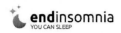

become more confident in your ability to handle whatever happens and be more okay with the possibility of sleeping poorly before a special event, even if it's challenging.

As you become less attached to sleeping well before special events, your nervous system will be much calmer at night, and you will come to sleep better before them. That being said, even normal sleepers sometimes experience sleep disruption before an early morning wake-up for a special event—so have realistic expectations for yourself.

END YOUR INSOMNIA FASTER

There's a lot to learn to master your insomnia. Whether you want support in learning to make peace with being awake or accountability in getting back to living fully as a way to decrease your sleep anxiety, we can help.

The course, coaching, and community of the End Insomnia Program offer the guidance, tools, and feedback you need to overcome your insomnia as quickly as possible. Getting results from the End Insomnia System takes work.

With coaching and implementation help and by becoming part of our solid community of people committed to the process of overcoming insomnia, we can make the journey easier for you and keep you on track.

There's a lot to learn to master your insomnia. For engaging video lessons and extra resources to help you master the knowledge and skills of this approach, join the End Insomnia Program.

The implementation tools and learning experiences we offer can speed up your learning and keep you on track through the ups and downs of overcoming insomnia.

CHECK IT OUT:

https://endinsomnia.com/program

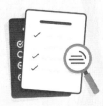

KEY CHAPTER TAKEAWAYS

☑   Work to reclaim your life if you've given up meaningful activities or goals to manage your insomnia. It's one of the best things you can do to move toward better sleep.

☑   Prove to yourself that you can live reasonably well regardless of how you sleep. Doing so lowers the stakes on sleep.

☑   Identifying and living by your **values** is a way to find meaning and fulfillment, even when dealing with fatigue, emotional burdens, and anxious thoughts. Connecting with your values can give you the motivation and resolve needed to face your day and reclaim your life from insomnia.

☑   Even if you feel groggy or low energy in the morning, don't assume you will feel bad the whole day. Notice how your energy fluctuates throughout the day, and work to build trust that you might get a second wind or feel better later, even if in the moment you feel quite low.

☑   When you find yourself dealing with **special event insomnia,** the stubborn increase in sleep anxiety before an event you want to feel rested for, the best thing to do is go through with it no matter how you sleep. If you can draw on the tools in this book to find more resilience, you can prove to yourself that you can handle special events, regardless of how you sleep—and you will gradually become less anxious about sleep before such events.

CHAPTER

13

Self-Compassion

Reducing the Sleep–Stopping Force Through Treating Yourself the Way You Would Treat a Loved One

We often don't treat ourselves the way that we treat others. In our inner dialogues, we can often be critical, cruel, or even abusive. Yet, judging or blaming ourselves when we are in emotional pain or in the midst of another bad night is not helpful.

Although self-criticism is extremely common, it's linked to negative mental health outcomes. A research review across 48 studies showed that self-criticism is associated with a range of mental health challenges, including depression, eating disorders, social anxiety disorder, personality disorders, and interpersonal problems.

So while we might feel that we are scolding ourselves into being more disciplined, doing better, or toughening up, critical self-talk instead leads to more shame, self-doubt, and frustration.

More "dirty pain."

The good news is we can intentionally change our self-talk with practice. Learning to have more kind and compassionate self-talk will help you suffer less—and cut out more of the dirty pain that makes insomnia so unbearable.

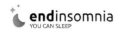

In fact, practicing self-compassion has been shown to decrease negative rumination (being stuck in a negative thought loop) and help the nervous system shift from fight-or-flight to a more restful state.

Self-compassion complements mindfulness and acceptance by inviting you to bring not only acceptance to your suffering but also open-hearted care and understanding.

It's easy to get angry and frustrated with yourself when you can't sleep. When you're stuck awake and miserable, you might harshly say things to yourself like, "Why is my body doing this to me? Why won't my thoughts just stop? What's wrong with me that I can't sleep like everyone else in the world?!"

One way to adopt a stance of greater kindness and understanding toward yourself is to remember that having insomnia is not your fault. The seed of doubt about sleep got planted in your mind. That was enough to start the cycle of anxiety. Your body started reacting to the sense of threat about not sleeping, and that made it even harder to sleep. It felt horrible, so the threat kept getting amplified. It's hard to get out once you're stuck in that cycle.

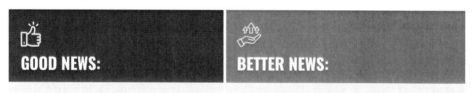

GOOD NEWS:

Insomnia is not a personal failing.

BETTER NEWS:

You have the power to break the cycle.

Anyone going through your situation with insomnia would be struggling. It's very difficult to get poor sleep consistently and to dread the night as a time of anxiety and misery rather than peaceful sleep. Recognizing that it's not your fault can help you be more gentle and understanding with yourself. You are in an objectively difficult and taxing situation. You deserve kindness.

The End Insomnia System works primarily by gradually lowering the perception of threat that has kept you awake. Research has shown that self-criticism and harsh self-talk amplify the activity in parts of your brain associated with threat, while practicing self-compassion lowers the activity of these regions.

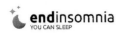
With these findings in mind, it is only practical to respond more gently to yourself when you are suffering and do your best to move away from harsh self-treatment.

SELF-COMPASSION EXERCISE 1: THE CARE YOU WOULD GIVE TO A FRIEND

Here is an exercise to try out self-compassion. First, think about a recent time you've suffered emotionally, with insomnia or something else. Now imagine that a good friend approached you and told you that they are going through that exact same thing. You really understand what it's like for them because you've been there too.

How would you treat that friend? What might you say to them? What actions might you offer them (sitting beside them, giving them a hug, etc.)? Rather than skipping over their pain to try to fix their problem, what words of support might you use to just let them know that you get it, that you feel for them as they go through this suffering, and that you care about them?

Once you think about the words or gestures you would offer to a friend, offer those same words or gestures to yourself. Take a moment and close your eyes, tap into your own struggle, and truly offer that care to yourself.

See what it's like to recognize your own pain and extend that warm-hearted support and understanding to yourself.

Although it might feel awkward at first, as with anything, you will get better with practice. In time, it can become much more natural to treat yourself with kindness and love, the way you would treat someone you really cherished.

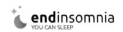

USING THE END INSOMNIA SYSTEM TO CHANGE YOUR RELATIONSHIP WITH YOURSELF - A STORY SELF-CRITICAL HIGH ACHIEVERS MAY RELATE TO

You may have been experiencing insomnia for months or years. You always pushed yourself in life and were proud of being able to meet your loved one's high expectations of you. But suddenly, you could barely function.

Now you find yourself experiencing relentless anxious and despairing thoughts at night... and intense physical symptoms of fatigue during the day. You may sometimes have full-blown anxiety attacks at night and then spend extra hours in bed in the morning to compensate.

Sleep became the central focus of your life. You likely withdrew from social engagements, cut down on work, and stopped doing other things that matter to you. Desperate for change, you likely tried a slew of treatments, perhaps even acupuncture, supplements, a range of routines and rituals, or even hiring a CBT therapist... all without seeing real change.

You couldn't see a way out of insomnia and began to feel like the life you had worked so hard to build was over... that your dreams and aspirations are forever unreachable because you feel incapacitated by insomnia. Based on the high expectations you hold for yourself, it's especially distressing how insomnia hijacked your life.

You likely see insomnia as a sign of weakness. While you didn't understand why you had insomnia, you may be deeply ashamed that you no longer feel like a strong and capable person. Like it was a personal failure that you could not overcome insomnia even when following expert advice.

Once you start applying the End Insomnia System, you'll take relief in understanding there's nothing fundamentally wrong with you—and that sleep anxiety is the issue. You'll implement a consistent sleep window to increase your sleep-starting force and begin to practice mindful acceptance to cut through some of your dirty pain. Your intense anxiety will begin to decrease.

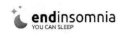
But even as your situation becomes a little more manageable, you may still worry your sleep might never return to normal. You're too hard on yourself, and on nights you sleep poorly, you may even feel like a failure. Since you so badly want to sleep normally again, when anxious thoughts start to spin at night, you may scold yourself with criticism and self-judgment for not being able to be calm.

Given the harsh judgments you direct toward yourself, using the system to learn self-compassion is critical. You'll come to understand that insomnia is not a sign of weakness or a personal failing. Soon, instead of defaulting to self-criticism, you'll practice being kind to yourself in your greatest moments of doubt, fear, and suffering. You'll begin to practice self-compassion during the day and become more mindful of when you criticize yourself. Though your tendency to automatically judge yourself won't immediately go away, in time, you'll begin to have access to self-kindness and be able to offer yourself more understanding and gentleness in times of need.

As you learn to be compassionate toward yourself, you'll become more capable of giving yourself what you may not have gotten a lot growing up - unconditional love and acceptance, even when you're struggling and vulnerable. In a way, you'll learn to be like a wise and loving parent (at least more of the time) toward the parts of yourself that feel scared, weak, and unworthy.

Learning to be kind and accepting toward yourself through the trial of insomnia will remove a lot of the unnecessary dirty pain you've been experiencing. As you combine self-compassion with the other tools in the End Insomnia System to increase your sleep-starting force and lower your sleep-stopping force, you'll begin to sleep better as your sleep confidence increases.

Before too long, you'll almost never experience sleep issues. When you occasionally do, it's not a big deal and your sleep gets back on track almost immediately.

Not only will you enjoy good sleep, but your relationship with yourself will transform through learning to be accepting and kind to yourself in times of vulnerability, even as you pursue ambitious goals.

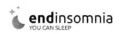
SELF-COMPASSION EXERCISE 2:
OFFERING YOURSELF
A CARING PHRASE

Here's a second exercise to practice self-compassion. First, bring to mind something that has recently caused you suffering or emotional heaviness, such as your sleep. Then try to tune in to where that emotional pain is held in your body. You might notice it as a tightness, a knot in your stomach, a heaviness in your chest, a numbness, a sense of emotion-laden fatigue in your body, or something else. Wherever you notice it, keep your attention on that feeling and then offer yourself some words of care. Try saying to yourself a phrase such as:

+ "I'm here for you. I see how much you're hurting right now. I care about you and I get it, this is really hard."
+ "May I open my heart to this suffering."
+ "May I treat myself with kindness."
+ "May I be gentle and understanding with myself."

Offering phases like this to yourself in a moment of suffering creates a softening in your relationship with yourself. Rather than judging, avoiding, or struggling against your emotional pain, you're acknowledging your pain and being there for yourself in a loving and accepting way. With practice, this brings soothing reassurance and can help you feel less alone in your most challenging times.

As a final note, being self-compassionate doesn't mean that you don't hold yourself accountable or that you give up on being disciplined. You can be kind to yourself and still make needed changes.

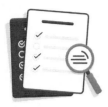

KEY CHAPTER TAKEAWAYS

☑   **Self-compassion** is the ability to respond to your own suffering and difficult moments with care, gentleness, and understanding.

☑   Judging, criticizing, or berating yourself when you encounter difficulties or can't sleep is not a helpful response. It just layers on more suffering and nervous system arousal.

☑   Self-compassion will help you reduce dirty pain and find more resilience in your journey through insomnia.

CHAPTER 14

Meditation

Reducing the Sleep–Stopping Force Through Developing a Daily Practice to Rebalance Your Nervous System

It is possible to train your nervous system to be calmer and less reactive. There are a variety of practices that can help recondition your nervous system— meditation, yoga, qi gong, tai chi—really, any practice that helps shift your body out of its habitual busy-doing state. The more often and more consistently we make this shift, the more our body learns it.

While the sleep knowledge you're learning in this book can help shift your experience, knowledge is usually not enough on its own. You need to combine multiple tools to create new experiences of resilience and calmness in the face of discomfort and uncertainty regarding your sleep. A nervous system regulation practice is one of those tools.

Mindfulness meditation is the daily practice we recommend for those using the End Insomnia System. Those who take up meditation tend to see better and faster results than those who do not. And a meditation practice is a great way to learn mindfulness and acceptance skills more deeply—and to bring more awareness and even-mindedness into all parts of your life.

Let's differentiate mindfulness from mindfulness meditation:

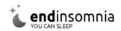

Mindfulness

Mindfulness is a skill you can practice anytime, anywhere, and doing anything. You just need to become intentionally aware of what's happening in the present moment and take an open and nonjudgmental stance toward whatever you notice (thoughts, feelings, senses, physical sensations).

Mindfulness meditation

Mindfulness meditation, however, is a formal and sustained practice of mindfulness.

When you meditate, you sit up straight with the intention to simply keep your attention in the present. Most commonly, this is done by keeping your attention on your breathing.

During meditation, your mind will inevitably wander many times. The idea is simply to *notice* when this happens and gently bring your attention back to your breath.

The point of mindfulness meditation is not to enter into a special calm and transcendent state. Rather, the point is to build a stronger capacity to be in the present moment and have more openness and even-mindedness toward whatever you notice. (You may often experience a downshifting of your nervous system into a calmer state during your meditation practice, but that's more a by-product than the goal.)

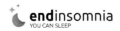

Three Reasons to Meditate for Long-Term Better Sleep

There are three primary reasons a daily mindfulness meditation practice will help you move toward overcoming your insomnia in the long term.

■ Reason 1: Meditation Helps Build the Mental Muscle of Present-Moment Awareness

As discussed in the chapter on mindfulness, awareness is a pivotal skill to reduce the amount of suffering you experience when you sleep poorly, and to cultivate less attachment to how you sleep night to night.

Being aware of what's happening in the present is the doorway to relating to your experience in new ways. Once aware, you can make intentional choices—including making beneficial changes that will help you overcome insomnia in the long term.

+ If you want to be more accepting, you first have to recognize that you're struggling.

+ If you want to be kinder to yourself, you must notice when you treat yourself harshly.

+ If you want to change unhelpful habits, you need to catch yourself in the moment and actively choose a new path—one that supports your sleep.

As you develop a meditation practice, the present moment becomes a trusted anchor to return to amid chaos, pain, and adversity. And by becoming more present more often, you also become more able to notice and savor the moments of life that are joyful and beautiful.

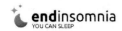

■ Reason 2: Mindfulness Meditation Helps Shift Your Nervous System Out of Fight-or-Flight Mode

The point of meditation is to learn to be more aware of and open to whatever is happening in your experience—not to force your experience to be different than it is. However, meditation does have a regulating effect on the nervous system.

Within your body, the **autonomic nervous system** is the part of your nervous system that controls involuntary processes in your body, like digestion, heart rate, breathing rate, and other organ functions. There are two branches within the autonomic nervous system: the **sympathetic** nervous system and the **parasympathetic** nervous system.

The *sympathetic nervous system* is responsible for turning on the fight-or-flight response (also known as the stress response). This is a very helpful response in certain situations but can also become chronically activated in an unhelpful way—as it is in the case of insomnia. The sympathetic nervous system is quick to turn on because our survival depends on being able to spring into action if danger suddenly appears.

The *parasympathetic nervous system,* by contrast, is responsible for helping your body shift into a state of safety, in which your body prioritizes rest, repair, and digestion. The parasympathetic nervous system's "rest and digest" response comes online much more gradually than the fight-or-flight response.

The sympathetic and parasympathetic nervous systems act in opposition to each other, meaning that when one is activated, the other is inhibited. With insomnia and other life situations that lead to chronic stress (and chronic perception of threat), the sympathetic nervous system over-functions.

This means that the parasympathetic nervous system under-functions—and the balance between these two nervous system branches is thrown off.

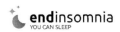

Mindfulness meditation practice has been shown by a substantial body of research to activate the parasympathetic nervous system's rest-and-digest response and turn down the sympathetic nervous system's fight-or-flight response.

While the point of meditation isn't to force calmness, with practice, meditation can become a reliable way to enter into a more calm state by activating your parasympathetic nervous system.

Having a daily practice that activates your parasympathetic nervous system can help you rest and recharge a little bit, even if you haven't had much sleep. Regular meditation practice also familiarizes your body and mind with how to switch out of fight-or-flight mode so that doing so becomes easier.

Although meditation can help downshift your nervous system, *do not try to use meditation to force yourself to sleep.* That would be a sleep effort, and sleep efforts do not work. As discussed in the chapter about what to do at night, it's fine to meditate at night if it helps you find more peace with being awake—so long as your intention is not to try to force sleep.

■ Reason 3: Mindfulness Meditation Can Change Your Brain in Helpful Ways

Mindfulness meditation practice maintained over several months can physically alter your brain in ways that can help you break the cycle of insomnia. A meta-analysis of over two dozen studies that used neuro-imaging scans to measure brain changes after an 8-week course of daily meditation found that meditation practice changed the brain in several positive ways.

These changes include increasing the connectivity and functionality of parts of the brain (such as the prefrontal cortex) responsible for rational thought and emotional regulation.

Daily meditation practice was also shown to decrease the size of the amygdala, the part of the brain responsible for activating the fight-or-flight stress response. So not only can meditation help you access awareness, acceptance,

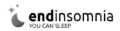

and emotional regulation in an immediate way, but it also can cause changes in the brain in the long term to make you naturally less reactive and more regulated.

Furthermore, a growing body of research suggests that a consistent daily mindfulness meditation practice alone is a viable treatment option for chronic insomnia.[,,]

This is not because meditation gives you a "trick to fall asleep," but rather because it helps break the stress overload cycle that drives insomnia. Meditation dials down your stress response and helps you be more accepting and less reactive.

Outside of helping you to overcome insomnia, daily mindfulness meditation practice has also been shown to improve general mental health, immune function, focus, and more. So it is worthwhile for the sake of general well-being as well.

You likely just want to get back to the life you had before insomnia ever started, so the idea of taking up a meditation practice may seem like an annoying "should." It may feel like it is just one more chore.

However, if you have ongoing insomnia, your nervous system is locked in a vicious cycle, and introducing a daily nervous system regulation tool like meditation can help break that cycle.

Meditation does take effort, but with time, it can grow to be a generally pleasant experience that helps you feel more centered and present in your day, even if you are fatigued. The effort of adding a meditation practice to your life is not a sleep effort. You're not doing it to control your sleep tonight. Rather, it's an effort aimed at long-term change.

When you meditate, you're making a consistent daily investment in regulating your nervous system and decreasing the amount of dirty pain you experience, so you suffer less and become less anxious about your sleep.

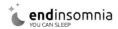

How to Meditate

I hope you are sold on the benefits of adopting a daily meditation practice as part of your long-term process of working through insomnia. Now, let's cover some basics about how to meditate.

In this form of meditation, you will be keeping your awareness anchored in the present moment. There are other forms of meditation in which you pay attention to body sensations or simply maintain an open awareness, but for now, focus on maintaining awareness of the sensation of your breath. This is both a simple and powerful practice.

- ✦ **Set a timer.** That will remove the need to check the clock (or at least remove the excuse to).
- ✦ **Sit with your spine straight,** rather than slouching or leaning back. This physically helps your mind stay sharp and alert.
- ✦ **Breathe using your diaphragm,** meaning your belly will expand on the inhale and fall on the exhale. This technique allows you to breathe more deeply and has a regulating effect on your nervous system. Once you're breathing into your belly, breathe at a normal and comfortable rate. Also, if possible, it's best to breathe through your nose rather than your mouth.

We also recommend you keep your eyes half-open, looking downward at a 45-degree angle toward the floor or wall in front of you. Keep your gaze soft; don't stare intently. Having your eyes partly open reduces the potential for daydreaming or drifting off to sleep.

It is completely normal for your mind to wander as you meditate. It happens to everyone. The key is to notice that your mind has wandered and then return your attention to your breath. That's it; just keep doing that until your timer goes off.

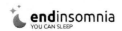

■ How Long to Meditate

There is value in even 3–5 minutes of meditation. Taking any amount of time out of your usual routine to slow down and breathe helps build the muscle of present-moment awareness; it also solidifies the intention to be more present in your day. A period of short meditation breaks the constant cycle of *going* and *doing* and *thinking*—it introduces your body and mind to the experience of just being.

Having a short but consistent daily meditation practice is better than occasionally meditating for longer periods. Consistency is required to change ingrained habits of mind and body.

While any amount of daily meditation is much better than no meditation, **20 minutes** per day is an ideal amount. This amount of time allows you to more fully switch out of the normal busyness of life—and taste a slower and more present way of being.

A daily practice of 20 minutes of meditation will also be enough to access the full range of benefits described earlier in this chapter. (You can build to 20 minutes gradually if it's too much at first.)

Meditation Apps: If you want help getting started, there are various apps that can help you build a meditation practice.

While it's fine to use an app to get started, it's best to transition into meditating without an app eventually. As you navigate difficult moments in life, you want to be confident that you can access your mindfulness skill set without a digital crutch.

Ready to reap the benefits? You have very little to lose by committing to a daily meditation practice, and you have much to gain. Although it may feel uncomfortable at first, or you may tell yourself your mind is too busy to meditate:

Anyone can meditate. Anyone can build the skill of being more aware and accepting of what's happening *now*.

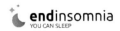

If you find that your mind is very active during meditation, that's totally fine. The practice will still benefit you. That's part of the beauty of it: Even if you constantly notice your mind wandering, and you have to bring your attention back to your breath again and again, you are still building the mental muscle of present-moment awareness.

GET REGULATED WITH US

Retraining your nervous system to be less reactive and more at ease takes work. If you're already feeling tired and starting up a new daily habit like meditation feels challenging, join the End Insomnia Program.

Our course, tools, coaches, and community can make adopting a meditation practice and doing everything else you're reading about in this book easier.

We'll support you in implementing these changes so you're not doing it alone and give you tools and guidance to make it as seamless as possible.

Additionally, being part of a community who are all using the same approach and working toward a common goal is a powerful way to make changes that would be difficult to make on your own.

We'd love to welcome you into our program and help you get your sleep issues worked out as soon as possible.

https://endinsomnia.com/program

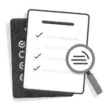

KEY CHAPTER TAKEAWAYS

☑ Mindfulness meditation is a sustained practice of mindfulness with several purposes:

  - To build the mental muscle of present-moment awareness in order to reduce dirty pain (unnecessary suffering) and build resilience.

  - To help shift your nervous system out of fight-or-flight mode.

  - To physically alter the brain (over time) to have a lowered threat response and greater access to calm and balanced thinking.

☑ Mindfulness meditation is not about attaining some transcendent state of mind; it is simply time you make to watch your breath and be in the present. It is taking time to stop *doing* and just *be*. In the process, you train your mind to be more aware, more accepting, and less reactive.

☑ Anyone can meditate. Although it takes effort to develop a daily meditation practice, it is an effort that will bring greater ease to your life and accelerate your journey through insomnia.

CHAPTER

15

Mindsets to Accelerate Your Progress

Reducing the Sleep-Stopping Force by Reframing Perceptions That Keep You Stuck—and Finding Empowerment Through Attitude Shifts

This chapter will cover a number of mindsets that are important to hold while on your journey to overcome insomnia. It's easier to make the changes required to end your insomnia when you are in a resilient, flexible, and empowered frame of mind.

Some of these ideas may be counterintuitive but bear with me. These mindset shifts can break mental loops that may be keeping you stuck.

The fastest way to change your situation is to change your mind.

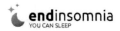

Adopt These Mindsets:

■ #1 You Are NOT an Insomniac

When you have insomnia, it's easy for it to become central in your life. It may feel like part of your identity. Your friends and co-workers may know you have trouble sleeping and ask about it regularly. Or perhaps you joke about how little you sleep or frequently talk about insomnia.

If having bad sleep has become part of your personal or social identity, you'll need to let that go. As you implement the End Insomnia System and progress toward a life without insomnia, identifying with insomnia will hold you back.

And if you ever refer to yourself as an insomniac, I recommend that you make a conscious effort to stop. You are not an insomniac. You are you. Insomnia is something you deal with—not who you are.

Talking about insomnia in casual conversations is generally not useful when working to improve your sleep. You're trying to make insomnia *less* of a big deal through this process—not *more* of one. Although it might feel good in the moment to vent about your poor sleep, generally speaking, the people you talk with are not really going to get what you're going through. Additionally, they may give you unsolicited, inaccurate, or unhelpful advice, which you are better off without.

In social settings, talk about the things you will talk about once your insomnia is totally gone. This is good practice for your life post-insomnia and will help you distance yourself from any "insomniac identity" you may be carrying.

There are better things to chat about socially than your sleep. If the people you used to talk with about insomnia ask about it, consider letting them know that you're in the process of addressing your insomnia, and part of that means not talking about it so much. You could also just say, "I slept fine," and leave it at that.

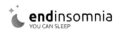

It's okay to continue to seek support—from a partner, close friend, or family member—with one condition: Make sure the person you're sharing with has some basic knowledge of the system you're using to overcome insomnia. Real support means encouragement and helpful reminders that facilitate your progress. If they don't understand how to best support you, they might say or do things that undermine the work you're doing.

I'll say more about how to get appropriate support from loved ones in the next chapter.

■ #2 Rough Nights and Tired Days Can Be a Positive Opportunity

When in the depths of insomnia, you may feel fear and helplessness at night and great dread as you face your mornings. You may feel totally at the mercy of insomnia. However, this can begin to change once you adopt a key mindset shift.

The mindset shift is this:

> If you want to become less anxious about not sleeping and the consequences, then it is on the nights you don't sleep well and the days you feel most tired that you have the most powerful opportunity to change.

When equipped with the right knowledge, tools, and perspectives, it becomes less threatening to face your fears. And when you face your fears and see that you can handle them, your fear naturally decreases.

The principle of overcoming anxiety by willingly facing your fears and becoming desensitized to the feared experience is the basis of exposure therapy, a foundational and evidence-based approach in mental health treatment.

Knowing that willingly facing your fears is the most direct and efficient way to overcome them, you can come to view the times you've most hoped to avoid

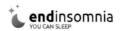

as actually an empowering opportunity to continue working through your insomnia.

You don't overcome sleep anxiety when everything is rosy, or you have a random good night but don't quite know why. You overcome sleep anxiety by making the thing you're afraid of less scary. You do this by facing what you've been dreading and realizing that it's no longer as scary now that you are equipped with the tools and knowledge of the End Insomnia System.

Seeing the opportunity in insomnia can apply to both the hard night and the day after.

Can you invite yourself to see a rough night as an opportunity to struggle less and build greater tolerance for being awake?

Can you view the next day as an opportunity to prove to yourself that you can get by—and maybe even have a great day?

■ #3 Bring Out Your Inner Rebel

As you make progress in working through your insomnia, keep an eye out for—and rebel against—any lingering sleep efforts that you continue to make, even subtly.

For example, you might still avoid certain foods or activities in the evening... or perhaps you still exercise during the day with the intention to make sleep happen that night.

Drawing on the confidence you've built through applying the knowledge and tools in this system, **rebel against any remaining self-imposed rules aimed at protecting you against the threat of poor sleep**. They don't help—and they actually undermine your progress by (1) reinforcing an insomnia identity, (2) causing a sense of deprivation that interferes with your quality of life, and (3) acting as sources of more anxiety.

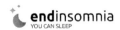

■ #4 Sleep Issues Are Not Responsible for Every Difficulty in Your Life

While you are rebelling against fixed ideas you may have, check to see if you are blaming insomnia for unrelated problems. Yes, having insomnia makes life a lot harder and can easily become a central preoccupation, but it's important to recognize that sleep issues are not responsible for every difficulty in your life.

When you're suffering from insomnia—especially when you've been experiencing it for a long time—it's easy to fall into the belief that if only insomnia were gone, life would be a breeze.

While it is true that life is easier without insomnia, it is also true that stress and difficult emotions are a normal and inevitable part of life.

Remember these two things: **First,** whether or not you have sleep issues, you will also likely face stress related to work, family, relationships, finances, anxieties about the future, or memories of things that have happened in the past. Even when you get past insomnia, life will still have its challenges. **Second,** such general life difficulties are likely partly responsible for some of the stress that you might currently be attributing to insomnia.

When you believe that your sleep issues are the only thing holding you back from a completely rosy life, that only increases the pressure to sleep. Remembering—and normalizing—that life will have stress even without sleep issues (and that such stressors may be part of your current distress) can help lower some of the unhelpful desperation to sleep.

■ #5 Find Moments of Gratitude

Just as insomnia is not responsible for every problem in your life, it does not negate every good thing in your life.

At times, you might become so consumed by managing your insomnia that it can be hard to zoom out and see the bigger picture. When bogged down by the burden of fatigue or anxiety, you might try taking a few moments to connect to a heartful sense of what you are grateful for.

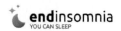

Remembering what is good in your life can offer perspective and a small dose of ease as you walk the path toward better sleep. Even dealing with insomnia, you may recognize that you are still grateful for things like your family, friends, work, the place you live, having food, or just that you are alive and able to experience this wild journey of being human.

While tapping into gratitude may not totally change your mood, it is another way to soften the sharp edge of rough nights and fatigued days.

■ #6 Be Patient

Don't rush through this book and expect that things will be totally different for you just because you read it. Overcoming insomnia takes patience, persistence, and learning to relate to difficulty in new ways.

Understanding what's going on with your sleep and learning how to overcome insomnia is a good start and can bring a good deal of relief in itself. However, to significantly reduce your sleep anxiety, you need to *apply* the practices and ideas of the End Insomnia System.

Knowing that you need to feel less anxious is not enough to lower your hyperarousal so you can sleep; only the *experience* of feeling less anxious can do that.

Applying the knowledge by practicing the tools you've learned will bring you that experience.

■ #7 Stick to the Plan Through the Ups and Downs

While the fatigue and emotional burden of insomnia may make it hard to stick to the plan, the alternative is staying stuck in insomnia.

This system requires a commitment to stay the course—even when you encounter doubts and obstacles.

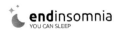

After a terrible night, an extra hard day, or a streak of tough nights, it's common to say something like, "This isn't working for me. I need to do something more radical. I need to change NOW."

It's important to remember that there are no quick fixes for insomnia. Even if you're doing everything right and applying the system in this book, sometimes things go off the rails.

Expect that. The best thing you can do is:

Trust the process.

Don't track your progress on a day-to-day basis. The End Insomnia system is an investment in long-term great sleep—not a quick-fix, one-night sleep effort.

The hard times will pass. Stick to the plan.

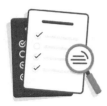

KEY CHAPTER TAKEAWAYS

☑ **You are not an insomniac.** Insomnia is something you deal with—not who you are. Let go of any ways insomnia has become part of your personal or social identity. Move away from talking about your sleep in social settings, as it won't help and will reinforce an "insomniac identity."

☑ **Insomnia is a golden opportunity.** A bad night or a day of fatigue is a powerful opportunity to work on overcoming fears by applying the tools you've learned to find more acceptance, calmness, and resilience.

☑ **Bring out your inner rebel.** Use your frustrations with insomnia to fuel your determination to let go of lingering sleep efforts and fear-based rules aimed at controlling your sleep. Rebelling against your self-imposed rules for sleep will ultimately lead to more ease at night.

☑ **Insomnia is not to blame for every issue in your life.** Challenges are a normal part of life, whether one has insomnia or not.

☑ **Find moments of gratitude.** Although dealing with insomnia is hard, it can be helpful to find moments of gratitude for what is good in your life. Doing so can help put the suffering of insomnia into perspective.

☑ **Be patient.** Have patience as you work through insomnia. This approach takes time. You must apply (not just read about) the skills and perspectives in this book in order to see real change. Knowledge about what's going on is helpful, but in order to lower your sleep anxiety, you need to experience being awake at night and dealing with the daytime consequences of insomnia in a less threatening way.

☑ **Stick to the plan.** The journey through insomnia has many ups and downs. Trust the process and stick to the plan even when you're struggling and having doubts.

16

Finding Appropriate Support

Whew! You've learned a lot!

There is just one more piece of the End Insomnia System—something that will make everything you are working on easier, faster, and (maybe even) more pleasant:

Find appropriate support.

Why Find Support?

Yes, you can go it alone. But many find their journey through insomnia is easier, faster, and less lonely with someone in their corner to cheer them on.

Having someone you can turn to who can offer some words of encouragement or help you think through what to do next is a huge relief if you've been trying to figure everything out on your own.

In times of struggle and doubt, the support of others can help you tap into greater hope, determination, and resilience. The journey of overcoming insomnia is easier when you don't feel alone.

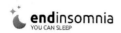

But for support to be helpful, it has to be appropriate. As I said in the last chapter, a loved one might—with the best of intentions—say or do something that will actually undermine the work you are doing.

For example, I don't encourage finding someone to just vent to about your insomnia—that will just reinforce any "insomniac identity" you might have.

Getting support is meant to help you stay on track through the hard times—and feel less isolated as you go through this process.

It's important to note that **you will not need support forever.** The idea behind getting support is not to become dependent on it—it's to facilitate and accelerate the process of overcoming insomnia.

An important test for whether the support you are getting is genuinely helpful: *It should make you feel more empowered, rather than dependent.*

■ How to Find Appropriate Support

Support in this process can come from many possible sources.

People in your life: First, it could come from a partner, family member, or friend. If you go this route, I recommend sharing this book with that person. They need to have a clear understanding of what you're going through—and the process of change that you're applying.

Your sources of support should understand the framework you are using to work through insomnia—the End Insomnia System. Otherwise, they might give feedback or advice that conflicts with what you are working on and adds more confusion to your experience.

Professional help: Second, support could come from a professional (such as a therapist) who can talk with you about what you're struggling with and help you stay on track in your journey through insomnia. Most therapists will not be familiar with the specific ideas in this system, but even just having someone empathetic to talk with can be helpful.

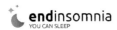

If you seek professional help, it would be a good idea to clearly outline the End Insomnia System so they know what you are working on. An easy way to do that is to share this book with them.

The End Insomnia Program: Third, you could join us at the End Insomnia Program. We've designed the program to provide:

+ Expert guidance and support to help you get unstuck and back on track when you feel lost and discouraged.

+ Community support from peers committed to overcoming insomnia and learning and applying the End Insomnia System alongside you.

+ Accountability tools to keep you focused on what needs to be done and give you the structure and incentive to make needed changes and progress toward better sleep.

+ An engaging video course to help deepen your understanding of the End Insomnia System—and turn that knowledge into a felt experience of transformation.

JOIN US AT:

https://endinsomnia.com/program

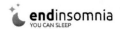

Times to Reach Out to Your Support System

Once you have a support system in place, use it:

- ✦ When you have a hard time.

- ✦ If you feel alone, lost, or overwhelmed by your insomnia experience.

- ✦ When you want to talk through a skill or idea you're applying that needs some fine-tuning.

- ✦ To recognize and reflect on the changes you've made—and how your experience is changing.

- ✦ To plan what to work on next.

- ✦ When you want encouragement—or accountability—to keep going forward.

Congratulations on learning the End Insomnia System! If you are feeling uncertain about any of it, or unsure about what to do next or how to do it... we've got you.

In Part 3, we'll pull together the ideas you've learned and answer some common questions. (And, of course, our program is always there for you.)

KEY CHAPTER TAKEAWAYS

☑ You will ease and accelerate your journey through insomnia if you have someone who understands your situation and can support you through the hard times and keep you on track in applying the system.

☑ Support could come from:

- Family or friends (share the book with them).

- A professional (such as a therapist).

- The **End Insomnia Program** (specifically designed for this purpose).

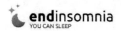

At the end of Part 2, I have a little 'ask' to make on behalf of everyone behind the End Insomnia System.

The only way for us at endinsomnia.com to accomplish our mission of helping the millions struggling with insomnia to sleep great is by reaching them.

And most people do judge a book by its cover (and its reviews).

If you have found this book valuable thus far, please take a brief moment and leave an honest review of the book and its contents on https://endinsomnia.com/review.

It will probably take less than 60 seconds, and your review will help:

- ✦ ...one more suffering individual sleep better soon
- ✦ ...one more spouse have a peaceful night
- ✦ ...one more person's life be free of insomnia

Thank you from the bottom of my heart.

YOU CAN LEAVE YOUR REVIEW BY FOLLOWING THE LINK:

https://endinsomnia.com/review

Yours,

Ivo

Part 3

Let's Sleep

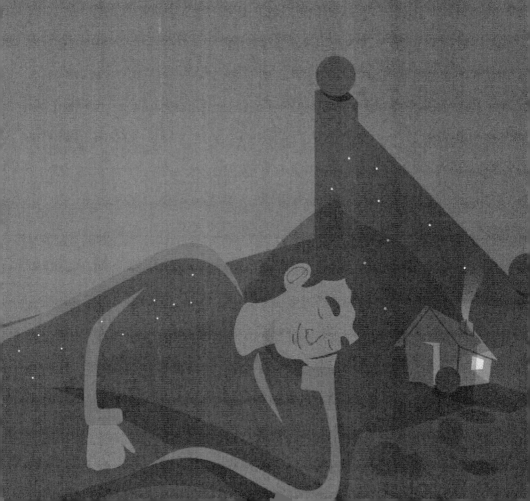

CHAPTER 17

Pulling It All Together

You've now learned the pieces that make up the End Insomnia System. This chapter will give a high-level overview of how all these pieces fit together. If you've been applying the ideas and exercises as you've read through the book, that's great.

If you have not or are looking for more guidance about how to prioritize what changes to make, this chapter will help you.

Here is a visualization of the End Insomnia System:

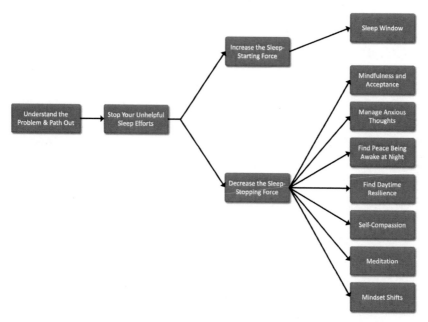

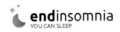

First, Ensure You Understand Insomnia—and the Path Out:

A difficult situation you understand and see a way through is less threatening than a difficult situation that you don't understand and feel completely powerless over. It's also important to eliminate misconceptions about insomnia, such as the myths that it will kill you or destroy your health.

It's important to remember that sleep anxiety is the primary root cause of most persistent insomnia. So reducing sleep anxiety—and the nervous system hyperarousal it causes—is the way to end insomnia permanently.

Stop Unhelpful Sleep Efforts

Remember: "Sleep efforts" are things you do to try to make sleep happen in the short term—and include sleeping pills and other substances, rigidly following sleep hygiene protocols, and rules and rituals aimed at trying to force sleep to happen on a given night.

Sleep efforts don't work. Sleep is a passive biological process that you cannot force to happen using willpower. Sleep efforts perpetuate sleep anxiety and undermine your confidence in your natural ability to sleep without any special effort.

Rather than making futile sleep efforts, you must instead focus on creating the conditions for effortless good sleep to happen on its own in the long term.

Review Chapters 2–7 to solidify your understanding of sleep, insomnia, and what you need to do to help your nervous system be sleep-compatible.

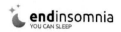

Sleep Is Controlled ONLY by the Sleep-Starting Force and Sleep Stopping Force

The journey to end your insomnia can be explained very simply:

1. Increase the sleep-starting force.
2. Decrease the sleep-stopping force.

The sleep-starting force consists of your sleep drive and your circadian rhythm. To increase your sleep-starting force, get your biology on your side by implementing a sustainable "sleep window"—the time you consistently set aside as your opportunity to sleep each night. Pair your sleep window with a low-pressure wind-down routine in the 45–60 minutes before bed.

Increasing your sleep-starting force ensures you have the highest probability of sleeping well each night, and also sets you up to rebuild sleep confidence in the long term.

Review Chapter 8 for guidance on how to use a sleep window to ensure you have a strong sleep-starting force at bedtime each night.

The sleep-stopping force consists of sleep anxiety and the hyperarousal it creates.

Entrenched sleep anxiety cannot be switched off overnight. To decrease your sleep-stopping force, you need to gradually work to reverse your sleep anxiety and the sense of threat your body feels at night. With time, you will retrain your nervous system to consistently be in a sleep-compatible state at night.

The End Insomnia System has many tools and strategies to help you suffer less when you sleep poorly, lower the stakes on sleep, and rebalance your nervous system.

Some of the tools you've learned include:

+   Mindfulness and acceptance.
+   Techniques for managing anxious thoughts.

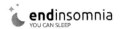

- ✦ Nighttime strategies to find peace when you can't sleep and break the hyperarousal cycle.

- ✦ Daytime strategies to lead a rich, full life even while you are working through your insomnia.

- ✦ Self-compassion.

- ✦ Meditation: a daily mindfulness meditation practice to build the skill of present-moment awareness and help recondition your mind and nervous system to be calmer and less reactive.

- ✦ Mindsets to help accelerate your progress.

- ✦ Finding appropriate support—empowering companionship and "help" that is genuinely helpful (and that does not inadvertently undermine your hard work).

You can review ways to lower your sleep-stopping force in Chapters 9–15.

Put It All Together, Piece by Piece

There is a lot to learn and weave together. You don't need to do everything at once. Work on the tools piece by piece at a pace that feels reasonable to you.

As you become more familiar with the tools, they will become less effortful and more automatic. With time and persistence, you will unlearn your sleep anxiety and conditioned hyperarousal and open yourself to great sleep on a consistent basis.

Remember, as you take steps to reduce the daytime consequences of insomnia, you will feel less anxiety at night. Likewise, when you learn to experience being awake at night with more acceptance and calm, you will experience fewer negative consequences during the day.

The actions you take to lower sleep anxiety in the day and the night are equally important.

KEY CHAPTER TAKEAWAYS

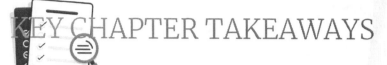

An overview of the components in the End Insomnia System:

- ☑ Understand insomnia—and the way out.
- ☑ Let go of sleep efforts.
- ☑ Increase your sleep-starting force by implementing a sleep window.
- ☑ Decrease the sleep-stopping force by learning to:
  - Suffer less through mindfulness and acceptance.
  - Manage anxious thoughts.
  - Find more peace and acceptance at night when you can't sleep.
  - Live fully during the day, even when you haven't slept well.
  - Regard yourself with self-compassion.
  - Develop mindsets that keep you on track.
  - Make the whole process easier by adopting a daily mindfulness meditation practice.
- ☑ Find support that empowers and helps you (and that doesn't undermine your hard work).
- ☑ The actions you take to reduce your sleep anxiety at night help you during the day. The actions you take to reduce your sleep anxiety during the day help you at night. Daytime and nighttime actions you take to help your situation are equally important.

CHAPTER

18

The Path to Sleep

In the last chapter, we did a quick refresher of the End Insomnia System as laid out in Part 2.

Now, let's discuss what the arc of change looks like as you put the End Insomnia System into practice.

While the journey through insomnia has ups and downs, there is a general set of phases that people go through as they use the End Insomnia System to overcome insomnia.

I call this the **Path to Sleep**.

Keep in mind that this trajectory is not fully linear: There may be times when you find yourself repeating phases—or you might identify with being in multiple phases at the same time.

As you read the descriptions, see which phases resonate for you. Notice—and give yourself credit for—any earlier phases you have now worked through.

Above all, view your process with self-compassion.

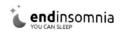

Phases of the Path to Sleep

■ Phase 1: Lost & Suffering

You've tried "everything" to fix your sleep—sleep hygiene, sleeping pills, lavender oil, weighted blankets, relaxation techniques, a hot bath or tea before bed, avoiding blue light before bed, making your room extremely dark, and countless other fixes. You are lost in confusion about what's happening with your sleep. You've tried so many things to fix it and have been disappointed. You are constantly googling the "solution" or watching endless Youtube videos to no avail.

You are afraid of getting your hopes up and being let down again. You are exhausted, depleted, and craving good sleep. You want good sleep more than anything, but as hard as you try, nothing seems to work. The situation feels out of control, your experience is hellish, and you are desperate for relief. You likely engage in many unhelpful perceptions, reactions, and behaviors that are part of what drives the vicious cycle of insomnia for you.

■ Phase 2: Finding Hope

Finding hope starts with proper education about insomnia—and the path out. You begin to understand why you have insomnia, that there's nothing uniquely wrong with you, and you see that there is a path to normal sleep. Your sleep hasn't improved much yet, but you feel some relief from understanding these ideas and beginning to apply them to change faulty perceptions.

■ Phase 3: Making Key Behavior Changes

You are letting go of unhelpful sleep efforts and implementing gentle changes in your sleep schedule and bedtime routine to optimize your natural sleep-starting force. You are facing the discomfort of letting go of old crutches and unhelpful behaviors. There can be some worsening of insomnia as you do

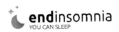

this, but it doesn't last—and you come to see that you can sleep even without engaging in habitual behaviors you may have thought you needed.

■ Phase 4: Experiencing Some Anxiety Reduction

You understand that you need to lower your fears of getting poor sleep in order to worry less and sleep better—but it's still difficult to really experience that. You are beginning to apply the tools in the End Insomnia System to lower your sleep-stopping force.

You are learning to work with your mind and body to find a more peaceful and accepting state in the day and the night. There are glimpses of the experience of greater calm and less fear, but still many ups and downs with your sleep— and times where it feels like you're not "getting it" when it comes to applying this approach.

You may doubt that this can work for you. The important thing here is to keep going.

You're reconditioning your nervous system to be less reactive and to feel safer at night—and that takes consistent practice in applying the various components of the End Insomnia System.

You're taking moments to be mindful and practice mindful acceptance during the day. Self-compassion is also reducing some of your struggles and helping you to be kind to yourself when things are hard.

You are also working to live more fully and let your deepest values guide your decisions, as opposed to the whims of your feelings. Meditation is another practice you are adopting to increase your mindfulness skills and as a long-term nervous system regulation tool.

Some conditioned hyperarousal symptoms may be lessening at this phase. You may begin to have times when you feel calm at night but still have trouble sleeping. It can take time for your body to learn that it's safe to let its guard

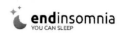

down and open up to sleep—but feeling calmer in bed is a big step on the path to get there. There can still be subtle layers of nervous system arousal that remain active even if you're feeling pretty calm. You will work through these layers with time.

■ Phase 5: Feeling Non-Attachment

As you maintain sleep-optimizing behaviors and continue to consistently practice the skills and mindsets of the End Insomnia System, you find over time that you are truly less worried about your sleep over time.

You are likely sleeping better more consistently, but there are times when your sleep is still pretty bad. However, in both the good and the bad times, you are experiencing a more durable sense of non-attachment, more confidence in yourself to handle whatever happens, and less fear about bad sleep and the consequences.

You are more tolerant of discomfort, you're calmer in situations that used to distress you, and you're consistently suffering less than you used to— even when tough nights happen. You know you can find meaning and even enjoyment in your day, even if you are fatigued.

Also, you are beginning to see a further reduction in conditioned hyperarousal symptoms, such as hypnic jerks, jolting wide awake from sleep, and drifting in and out of light sleep.

You probably don't have perfect non-attachment to how you sleep, but you don't need to. Just having a good amount of non-attachment is enough to lead to major positive changes in your sleep. At this point, you have strong confidence in this path to overcome insomnia because you have experienced the changes it brings.

You are willing to keep walking this path for however long it takes and are seeing the benefits of using the skills of this system in other parts of your life.

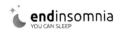

The phase of feeling true non-attachment is the most important one to reach—but getting there can take longer than the other phases. This is especially likely if you have had insomnia for many years, if insomnia has felt especially traumatic, or if you have other major anxieties and stressors in your life that you're dealing with at the same time.

This program is aimed at helping you get to non-attachment—because once you arrive, good sleep is not far behind.

Also, it's important to recognize that although we're calling out feelingnon-attachment as a landmark of this phase, greater non-attachment to your sleep is something you're cultivating and building toward in all phases of your journey, not just this one.

One final thing you might experience in this phase (or possibly later) is feeling more exhausted and fatigued in the day, even if you sleep better. This is a common experience and happens because your body is beginning to shift out of survival mode—so there is more space for you to feel the fatigue that's been buried under the anxiety and hyperarousal. Know that this is normal and will pass as you keep moving forward and your nervous system recalibrates to a state of greater safety and calm.

■ Phase 6: Consistently Sleeping Better

Consistent good sleep follows from a sleep-compatible nervous system. You've arrived at a place of less fear and less nervous system agitation around sleep, and you truly don't feel much attachment to whether you sleep well or not because you are confident you can handle whatever happens. As a result, you are consistently sleeping better. You did it!

You feel gratitude for good sleep and relief that insomnia is fading from your life. Hyperarousal symptoms in the day and night continue to lessen as your body and unconscious mind more fully get the message that it is safe and there is no threat. You may still have some worries about insomnia returning, especially before some special event that you want to be well-rested for.

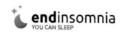

■ Phase 7: Building Further Confidence—and Working Through Setbacks

Even when you're consistently sleeping better, a part of you worries about the possibility of insomnia returning. Though things are much better, your mind may hold onto memories of great suffering or traumatic experiences regarding your sleep in the past.

Sometimes a setback happens. You have a night or a few nights of worse sleep. Maybe it was triggered by special event anxiety. It also might have been triggered by remembering how horrible your sleep used to be and doubting that you've truly overcome your insomnia.

When you have a setback, it's like a little pocket of fear that has been holding on inside of you is bubbling up to the surface. This is an opportunity to process and permanently release it.

As you face the setback by reapplying the skills you've learned and proving to yourself how much you've changed, you realize more fully that you don't need to be afraid anymore—and good sleep returns before long.

In the process, you've had the vitally important experience of becoming even less afraid of poor sleep and less afraid of any future setbacks. As you go through the process of having setbacks and then regaining confidence, these setbacks happen less and less until they almost never happen. Anxiety about whether you will sleep well before special events also fades.

■ Phase 8: Life Beyond Insomnia

You are fully over your insomnia. You don't think about sleep anymore; it is just a normal part of life. You sleep well the vast majority of the time; it is restful and enjoyable.

There are times when you experience occasional bad nights, especially under stress, because this is a normal part of being human, and it happens to

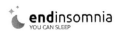

everyone. However, you are not distressed or afraid when this happens and can go with the flow.

An occasional bad night can no longer spiral into ongoing insomnia—because you've changed. You have changed in ways that prevent insomnia from being able to take root again. You are not afraid. You get to focus on living and enjoying your life. You look back at your journey through insomnia and feel proud of yourself for overcoming such a challenge. The journey through insomnia has taught you many things about yourself and helped you become a person with greater awareness, courage, resilience, and tenacity—all traits that you will carry with you for the rest of your life.

You can do this. Many have walked this path before you and are now fully past their insomnia and enjoying life with good sleep. If you follow the system in this book and apply yourself fully, you can experience big changes and gradually attain consistent restorative sleep. It's only a matter of time.

The Timeline to Restore Your Sleep

It is very natural to wonder how long this process will take. As I said earlier in the book, there is no guaranteed timeline for getting results from this system. The speed of change can vary from person to person based on a variety of factors.

The best practice is to let go of the timeline. The more closely you monitor your progress, the more anxiety you're going to feel about sleep and the process of overcoming insomnia. Make your intention to just take it one day at a time. Try to appreciate the journey of learning, making changes, and developing new skills.

While it's not easy, the more patient you can be in the process, the better. Letting go of the timeline is actually an embodiment of the attitude of non-attachment that will help you release your anxiety—and open up to better sleep.

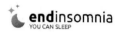

There will be times you feel like hell and periods when you want to give up. To see results, you have to keep going and trust the process. The hard times pass, and things even out.

This path takes work and commitment, but it can reward you with what you want more than anything: great sleep on a consistent basis—and freedom from ever worrying about your sleep again.

There is a lot to learn and put into practice in order to overcome insomnia, but you don't need to do it alone.

Join the **End Insomnia Program** to speed up the process. You'll get your questions answered, receive guidance from our coaches, and have accountability in making important changes. You'll also become part of our supportive and positive community of people with shared experiences working toward the shared goal of an insomnia-free life. We'll be there for you through the ups and downs.

GO HERE TO GET STARTED:

https://endinsomnia.com/program

KEY CHAPTER TAKEAWAYS

☑ Reference the phases in the Path to Sleep laid out in this chapter to assess where you are in the process of overcoming insomnia, and to see what lies ahead.

☑ Although it's natural to want to know the exact timeline for a return to better sleep, the best practice is to let go of the timeline. Take it day by day and focus on increasing the sleep-starting force while lowering the sleep-stopping force.

CHAPTER

19

Managing Setbacks

As you apply the End Insomnia System over time, know that setbacks are an inevitable—and even necessary—part of fully reversing insomnia.

It's wonderful to start sleeping better more consistently after struggling with insomnia. There can be an enormous sense of relief as you come to trust in your sleep, and you find that sleep is less and less on your mind. However, I've rarely seen someone completely overcome insomnia without having a few setbacks along the way.

Setbacks—and Solutions

Here are three common scenarios:

■ Setback Scenario 1:

First, setbacks can happen because you get **attached** to your improved sleep: *Attachment rekindles sleep anxiety.* You're enjoying better sleep, it's exactly what you wanted, but then you begin to fear the possibility that you could lose it again. You think back on your past sleep struggles, and you do NOT want to go back there. Even if you had previously found less attachment to your sleep and a true willingness to tolerate whatever happens, as you get more attached to sleeping well, old fears of poor sleep begin to arise and create sleep performance anxiety.

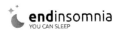

This performance anxiety may then trigger a setback where you find yourself temporarily sleeping poorly again.

■ Setback Scenario 2:

Second, as you work through your insomnia, you may experience a vulnerability to setbacks around special events. A **special event** could be a social gathering, travel, or a big day at work the next day. Even if you have been sleeping pretty normally, suddenly, you begin to worry more about your sleep because you want to be sure you are at your best for the special event. Your sleep anxiety rises, and then you have a harder time sleeping. Sometimes, this can lead to a stretch of poor nights as you fall back into old habits and begin feeling again under threat from insomnia.

■ Setback Scenario 3:

Third, you might encounter a **seemingly inexplicable** setback. In fact, this apparently random experience is likely a resurgence of old conditioned hyperarousal.

After all, your nervous system held that association of night with threat for a long time. Sometimes the old wiring will re-fire even when it doesn't feel like you've done anything to activate it. You might find yourself struggling to sleep and feel frustrated because your body seems to be sabotaging your good progress. This can lead to a period of worse sleep as old worries and unhelpful behaviors reemerge.

■ The Setback Solution

Regardless of what brought it on, **the solution to any setback is the same**: Reapply the knowledge and tools to *raise* your *sleep-starting force* and *lower* your *sleep-stopping force*.

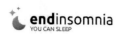

Though it's distressing to fall back into a bout of bad sleep after you've experienced the relief of good sleep, the best thing you can do is to keep working to care less about how you sleep.

By reapplying the system, you remind yourself, "Oh yeah, when I keep the right perspective and show up in the right ways, this really is not so unbearable." You remember that you truly do have control over your insomnia when you take a long-term approach using the tools of the End Insomnia System.

With all this in mind, remember that setbacks are an inevitable part of the journey. When you expect that setbacks will occur, you will be less crushed and confused when they happen. You can respond to them intentionally to get back on track as quickly as possible. If you've reached a state of lower sleep anxiety once, you can do it again.

Not only are setbacks an inevitable part of the process, but they are also *necessary* for truly overcoming insomnia. Setbacks are the way that lingering layers of sleep anxiety are purged from your system. If you never had a setback, you would likely think back on the idea of your insomnia returning with a sense of fear and dread.

However, when you start sleeping better and then have a setback, you are forced to learn again that when you approach insomnia with the right tools, it's not as scary or debilitating as you remember. Each time this happens, you become less and less afraid of insomnia going forward.

The process of setbacks strengthening your confidence continues until you truly are *not afraid* of sleeping poorly and you trust that sleep will happen for you.

As you reach this place of confidence in and non-attachment to your sleep, you will no longer experience insomnia—because your nervous system has no reason to keep you up at night.

KEY CHAPTER TAKEAWAYS

☑   Setbacks are an inevitable part of the process of overcoming insomnia. Expect them to happen. Having a setback does not mean you are back to square one.

☑   While setbacks can occur for many reasons, the solution is *always* to continue applying the skills and information to lower sleep anxiety and set the stage for good sleep in the long term.

☑   Be careful of reverting to old unhelpful behaviors or mindsets during a setback. While it's tempting to revert to using old sleep efforts, you have to let go of trying to control your sleep in the short term because it doesn't work.

☑   Setbacks are *necessary* to fully address your insomnia. Setbacks help you process and release additional layers of fear and conditioning around your sleep. Setbacks become less and less common as you learn more fully that you no longer need to be so afraid of poor sleep and that you can handle whatever happens.

Conclusion

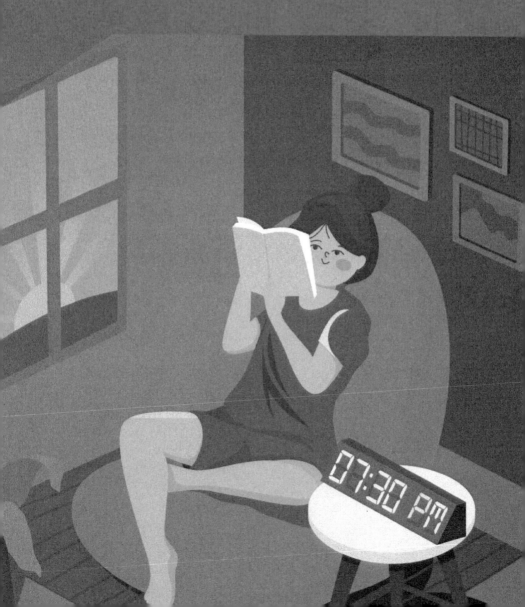

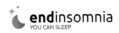

Congratulations!

You've now learned the End Insomnia System.

I hope you've begun to apply what you are learning and are seeing some positive changes.

If you're not there yet, keep it up. With time, you can achieve the good sleep you are seeking.

Remember, there is no overnight solution for insomnia. Overcoming insomnia is a long-term process of learning how to be calmer in the midst of discomfort and reconditioning your nervous system to be sleep-compatible at night.

If you stick with it, the End Insomnia System can carry you through to the dawn of a new chapter of your life.

Additionally, it's helpful to remember the tools you are learning to handle the deep distress of insomnia *apply to all of life*. By internalizing and practicing these skills, you will not only reclaim great sleep, but you will also better navigate the inevitable challenges of life with greater even-mindedness, resilience, and wisdom.

This book gives you the tools to overcome your insomnia—but it is still a hard road. The journey can be made more quickly and easily with support.

If you decide you want help through this process, join the **End Insomnia Program**.

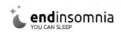

You'll get access to:

- ✦ An engaging video course to help you put the system into practice in your life and accelerate your journey through insomnia.

- ✦ Tools to track your implementation, provide accountability, and discover what you need to focus on when you feel lost or like you've plateaued in your progress.

- ✦ Weekly group coaching calls to help you through your sticking points and learn from the progress of others.

- ✦ A supportive online community on the same journey as you. This community supports one another through the tough times and celebrates the successes as you move step-by-step toward effortless, anxiety-free sleep.

JOIN US HERE:

https://endinsomnia.com/program

The coaches at the End Insomnia Program have personally known the pain of insomnia and have successfully overcome it. You deserve to live life without carrying the constant burden of insomnia. We can help.

To fearless sleep,

Ivo

P.S. I have one final ask:

If you have found this book useful in understanding your sleep issues or if it has given you hope and new tools to shift your experience, then please take 60 seconds right now to leave an honest review on endinsomnia.com/review

It will only take a minute on your part, and your review will help this knowledge reach more people struggling with sleep and feeling lost and discouraged about what to do.

Your feedback can help people in need reclaim their lives from poor sleep and find the energy and inspiration to live well.

If you know someone in your life who struggles with sleep, please send them this book so they can benefit too.

– Thank you!

YOU CAN LEAVE THE REVIEW HERE ON:

https://endinsomnia.com/review

Endnotes

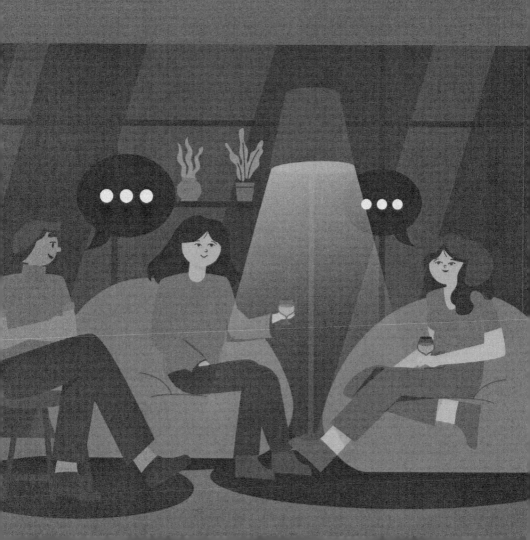

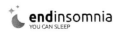

1. Li, S. B., Borniger, J. C., Yamaguchi, H., Hédou, J., Gaudilliere, B., & de Lecea, L.(2020). Hypothalamic circuitry underlying stress-induced insomnia and peripheral immunosuppression. *Science advances, 6(37)*. https://doi.org/10.1126/sciadv.abc2590

2. *What's so great about acceptance and commitment therapy?* (2022, March 22). Psychology Today. https://www.psychologytoday.com/us/blog/the-art-self-improvement/202203/whats-so-great-about-acceptance-and-commitment-therapy

3. Dindo, L., Van Liew, J. R., & Arch, J. J. (2017). Acceptance and Commitment Therapy: A Transdiagnostic Behavioral Intervention for Mental Health and Medical Conditions. *Neurotherapeutics : the journal of the American Society for Experimental NeuroTherapeutics, 14(3)*, 546–553. https://doi.org/10.1007/s13311-017-0521-3

4. arskadon, M. A., Dement, W. C., Mitler, M. M., Guilleminault, C., Zarcone, V. P., & Spiegel, R. (1976). Self-reports versus sleep laboratory findings in 122 drug-free subjects with complaints of chronic insomnia. *The American journal of psychiatry, 133(12)*, 1382–1388. https://doi.org/10.1176/ajp.133.12.1382

5. Edinger, J. D., & Fins, A. I. (1995). The distribution and clinical significance of sleep time misperceptions among insomniacs. Sleep, 18(4), 232–239.https://doi.org/10.1093/sleep/18.4.232

6. Trimmel, K., Eder, H. G., Böck, M., Stefanic-Kejik, A., Klösch, G., & Seidel, S. (2021). The (mis)perception of sleep: factors influencing the discrepancy between self-reported and objective sleep parameters. *Journal of clinical sleep medicine : JCSM : official publication of the American Academy of Sleep Medicine, 17(5)*, 917–924. https://doi.org/10.5664/jcsm.9086

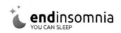

7.   Borkovec, T. D., Lane, T. W., & VanOot, P. H. (1981). Phenomenology of
        sleep among insomniacs and good sleepers: wakefulness experience
        when cortically asleep. Journal of abnormal psychology, 90(6), 607–
        609.
        https://doi.org/10.1037//0021-843x.90.6.607

8.   Mercer, J. D., Bootzin, R. R., & Lack, L. C. (2002). Insomniacs'
        perception of wake instead of sleep. Sleep, 25(5), 559-566.
        https://doi:10.1093/sleep/25.5.559

9.   Chang, A. M., Aeschbach, D., Duffy, J. F., & Czeisler, C. A. (2015).Evening
        use of light-emitting eReaders negatively affects sleep, circadian
        timing, and next-morning alertness. Proceedings of the National
        Academy of Sciences of the United States of America, 112(4), 1232–
        1237.
        https://doi.org/10.1073/pnas.1418490112

10.   *How much sleep do you really need?.* (2020, October 1). Retrieved from
        https://www.thensf.org/how-many-hours-of-sleep-do-you-really-
        need/

11.   Lovato, N., & Lack, L. (2019). Insomnia and mortality: A meta-analysis.
        Sleep medicine reviews, 43, 71–83.
        https://doi.org/10.1016/j.smrv.2018.10.004

12.   Loannidis J. P. (2005). Why most published research findings are false.
        PLoS medicine, 2(8), e124.
        https://doi.org/10.1371/journal.pmed.0020124

13.   Kircanski, K., Lieberman, M. D., & Craske, M. G. (2012). Feelings into
        words: contributions of language to exposure therapy. *Psychological
        science, 23*(10), 1086–1091.
        https://doi.org/10.1177/0956797612443830

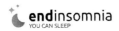

14. Brickman, P., Coates, D., & Janoff-Bulman, R. (1978). Lottery winners and accident victims: Is happiness relative?. *Journal of Personality and Social Psychology, 36*(8), 917-927.
https://doi.org/10.1037/0022-3514.36.8.917

15. Lyubomirsky, S., Sheldon, K. M., & Schkade, D. (2005). Pursuing happiness: The architecture of sustainable change. *Review of General Psychology, 9*(2),111–131.
https://doi.org/10.1037/1089-2680.9.2.111

16. Ekers, D., Webster, L., Van Straten, A., Cuijpers, P., Richards, D., & Gilbody, S.(2014). Behavioural activation for depression; an update of meta-analysis of effectiveness and sub group analysis. *PloS one, 9*(6), e100100.
https://doi.org/10.1371/journal.pone.0100100

17. Werner, A. M., Tibubos, A. N., Rohrmann, S., & Reiss, N. (2019). The clinical trait self-criticism and its relation to psychopathology: A systematic review -Update. *Journal of affective disorders, 246*, 530–547.
https://doi.org/10.1016/j.jad.2018.12.069

18. Kirschner, H., Kuyken, W., Wright, K., Roberts, H., Brejcha, C., & Karl, A. (2019). Soothing your heart and feeling connected: A new experimental paradigm to study the benefits of self-compassion. *Clinical Psychological Science, 7*(3), 545–565.
https://doi.org/10.1177/2167702618812438

19. Doerig, N., Schlumpf, Y., Spinelli, S., Späti, J., Brakowski, J., Quednow, B. B., Seifritz, E., & Grosse Holtforth, M. (2013). Neural representation and clinically relevant moderators of individualised self-criticism in healthy subjects. *Social Cognitive and Affective Neuroscience, 9*(9), 1333-1340.
https://doi.org/10.1093/scan/nst123

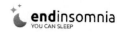

20.   Kim, J. J., Parker, S. L., Doty, J. R., Cunnington, R., Gilbert, P., & Kirby, J. N. (2020). Neurophysiological and behavioural markers of compassion. *Scientific Reports, 10*(1). https://doi.org/10.1038/s41598-020-63846-3

21.   Amihai, I., & Kozhevnikov, M. (2015). The influence of Buddhist meditation traditions on the autonomic system and attention. *BioMed Research International, 2015,* 1-13. https://doi.org/10.1155/2015/731579

22.   Tang, Y., Ma, Y., Fan, Y., Feng, H., Wang, J., Feng, S., Lu, Q., Hu, B., Lin, Y., Li, J., Zhang, Y., Wang, Y., Zhou, L., & Fan, M. (2009). Central and autonomic nervous system interaction is altered by short-term meditation. *Proceedings of the National Academy of Sciences, 106*(22), 8865-8870. https://doi.org/10.1073/pnas.0904031106

23.   Wu, S., & Lo, P. (2008). Inward-attention meditation increases parasympathetic activity: A study based on heart rate variability. *Biomedical Research, 29*(5), 245-250. https://doi.org/10.2220/biomedres.29.245

24.   Gotink, R. A., Meijboom, R., Vernooij, M. W., Smits, M., & Hunink, M. M. (2016). 8-week mindfulness based stress reduction induces brain changes similar to traditional long-term meditation practice – A systematic review. *Brain and Cognition, 108,* 32-41. https://doi.org/10.1016/j.bandc.2016.07.001

25.   Black, D. S., O'Reilly, G. A., Olmstead, R., Breen, E. C., & Irwin, M. R. (2015). Mindfulness meditation and improvement in sleep quality and daytime impairment among older adults with sleep disturbances: a randomized clinical trial. *JAMA internal medicine, 175*(4), 494–501. https://doi.org/10.1001/jamainternmed.2014.8081

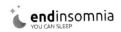

26. Gross, C. R., Kreitzer, M. J., Reilly-Spong, M., Wall, M., Winbush, N. Y., Patterson, R., Mahowald, M., & Cramer-Bornemann, M. (2011). Mindfulness-based stress reduction versus pharmacotherapy for chronic primary insomnia: A randomized controlled clinical trial. *Explore, 7*(2), 76-87. https://doi.org/10.1016/j.explore.2010.12.003

27. Ong, J. C., Manber, R., Segal, Z., Xia, Y., Shapiro, S., & Wyatt, J. K. (2014). A randomized controlled trial of mindfulness meditation for chronic insomnia. *Sleep, 37*(9), 1553–1563. https://doi.org/10.5665/sleep.4010

28. *The science of mindfulness.* (2020, September 7). Mindful. https://www.mindful.org/the-science-of-mindfulness/

29. Rauch, S. A., Eftekhari, A., & Ruzek, J. I. (2012). Review of exposure therapy: A gold standard for PTSD treatment. *The Journal of Rehabilitation Research and Development, 49*(5), 679. https://doi.org/10.1682/jrrd.2011.08.0152

Made in United States
North Haven, CT
03 August 2024

55681721R00124